From the Patients

"Since having my mercury fillings replaced, I noticed an increase in my energy level, and within six months the mental fog I consistently had was replaced by a clarity of thinking I hadn't experienced in years. Prior to the procedure, I suffered from extreme fatigue. My life and health have changed dramatically for the better!"   M. Uss

"I'd been plagued for years with symptoms that moved around my body - essentially structural (requiring chiropractic adjustments) and left-sided migraines. In the nearly three years since I had the mercury removed from my mouth, I have seen a gradual definite decline of these symptoms. Headaches are few and far between, and not severe (the old ones lasted three days) and my visits to a chiropractor are as-needed, and that now means every other month or less. In the old days, I'd locate chiropractors before travel. Now I don't even think about it."   V. Fulton

"I chose to have all my mercury amalgam fillings removed because I developed multiple chemical sensitivity. Once the fillings were removed, my chemical sensitivities in general lessened. In particular, I noticed that the muscle tension in my jaw, which I had for years, disappeared." P. Wolff, M.S., R.N.C.S.

"After struggling for years to recover from knee surgery, I had all of the amalgam fillings in my mouth replaced in 1992. Not only did I experience a remarkable improvement in my injured knee, but I also encountered a significant reduction in headaches, unexplained skin disorders and allergies (all of which had started about the time I first had amalgam fillings placed in my mouth). I have had only excellent experiences with "whole body dentistry" and gained an overall, improved sense of well being." T. LeVine

"I was being treated for different medical problems including hypothyroidism, irregular menstrual cycles and fatigue. After having my root canal tooth extracted, in the next month my cycles regulated - something that had not occurred in over ten years - and I stopped taking the hormone and thyroid medication. My energy level has improved and I am feeling better that I have in a long time!" J. Williams

"Since removing my amalgam fillings last winter, I have noticed a remarkable improvement in my digestion, specifically with regard to my tolerance of dairy products, and notably, though perhaps odd - bananas, which for the first time in years I am eating without getting a stomachache. Additionally, my skin is like a new friend - for the first time in uncountable winters, I have not experienced the painfully dry skin and eczema that have typically afflicted me during this season. Both of these results were unexpected benefits that I attribute to removing the amalgam fillings and detoxing the heavy metals from my system. Thank you for providing this option in health care, and keep up the good work." K. Mitchell

"Because I was having unexplained neurological symptoms and Dr. Breiner's examination indicated there was a lot of electrical activity in my mouth, I decided to have my amalgam fillings removed and replaced with other materials. The fuzziness I had been experiencing on almost a daily basis disappeared during the course of my four appointments. The lack of feeling and strength in my feet and hands took a little longer to go away completely, In addition, a highly welcome and completely unexpected thing occurred I didn't get sick that winter, not a cold or sore throat, nothing. That continued for the next six years. I can't help but believe that somehow the amalgam fillings were interfering with my immune system as well. Getting rid of those fillings was one of the best things I ever did for myself!" A. Levy

WHOLE-BODY DENTISTRY™

WHOLE-BODY DENTISTRY™

Mark A. Breiner, D.D.S.,F.A.G.D., F.I.A.O.M.T.

Discover the missing piece to better health

INTRODUCTION
by
Dr. Robert C. Atkins, M.D.

Quantum Health Press, LLC

Disclaimer Note to the Reader:

Although the author and publisher have exhaustively researched all sources to ensure the accuracy and completeness of the information contained in this book, we assume no responsibility for errors, inaccuracies, omissions or any inconsistency herein. Any inaccurate characterizations of people, places or organizations are unintentional.

The information and procedures contained in this book are based on the research and the personal and professional experience of the author. This book has been published for information and reference uses only. It is not intended in any respect as a substitute for a visit to a qualified dentist, physician, or other licensed health care practitioner. Every individual is genetically different, and no method of treatment is useful for everyone. If you have a dental or medical problem, please consult a qualified dentist, physician or health care provider for diagnosis and treatment under their supervision. The publishers and author are not responsible for any adverse effects or consequences resulting from the use of any suggestions, procedures, techniques, protocols, remedies or preparations discussed in this book.

Quantum Health Press, LLC
P.O. Box 1637, Fairfield, CT 06432
Tel: 203.396.0342; Tel. 888.277.1328(Orders); Fax: 203.372.5773

visit website for Whole-Body Dentistry™ at www.WholeBodyDentisty.com

0 2 0 1 0 0 9 9 / 9 8 7 6 5 4 3 2 1

If you are unable to order this book from your local bookseller, you may order directly from Quantum Health Press, LLC.

Quantity discounts available through publisher

DEDICATION

To my wife, Mona, a true woman of valor. Without her love and support, I could not do what I do.

To my sons, Adam and Justin, who have become outstanding young men.

And to my parents, Mickey and Rose, who have always been there for me.

ACKNOWLEDGMENTS

I would like to express my gratitude to those from whom I have learned, either in person or through their published works. Those names are too numerous to list in full. Among them are a few that have had a profound effect on me as a dentist. They are: Dr. Weston Price, Dr. Melvin Page, Dr. L.D. Pankey, Dr. Boyd Haley, Dr. Reinhard Voll, Dr. Dietrich Klinghardt, Dr. Michael Ziff, Dr. Murray Vimy, Doug Lieber, Sam Queen and Walter "Jess" Clifford.

I would like to single out Dr. Hal Huggins for his courage to speak the truth about amalgams, fluoride and root canals. With determination, perseverence and thirst for the truth, he has led the battle to change dentistry as it is commonly practiced. Every leader I know in the field of mercury toxicity has been influenced by Dr. Huggins.

Special acknowledgment to my colleagues and friends in the International Academy of Oral Medicine and Toxicology - a unique group of scientific truth seekers. Also to the members of DAMS, who support us professionals with tireless effort in helping to educate the public about amalgam, fluoride, etc. I am also indebted to my staff - Jane Wolinsky, Jennifer Duke and Dawn Basso for their support of me and all those who come to us for treatment. Thank you to Attorney Charlie Brown for his dedication to the cause and to Attorney Rick Ferris for his expertise and friendship. Thanks to my son, Justin Breiner, for his art work, to Jim Saslo of Northeastern Press for all his help above and beyond the scope of "printer", and to Barbara and Harold Levine for sharing their publishing know-how. Thank you to my best friend, Bob Wolinsky, for being all that a friend needs to be. A final acknowledgment and thank you to Dr. Robert Atkins and Dr. Warren Levin and to my patients who graciously wrote about their experiences so that others might benefit.

FOREWORD

My rheumatoid arthritis was diagnosed in 1993 when I was 26 years old. My initial symptoms included: chronic fatigue, a weight gain of 40 pounds, emotional stress, mood swings, sleeplessness, hair loss - in addition to the weakness, swelling and joint pain that are general indicators of the disease.

I sought the most aggressive treatment available at the Hospital for Special Surgery since they were the number one ranked rheumatology center in the country. I had sporadic relief from traditional arthritis medications, but results were short-lived. A medication would have a positive result and then its effectiveness would diminish, often ending in an allergic reaction or a super flare up of the arthritis. After trying all available arthritis drugs I turned to homeopathic medicine. Results were amazing, but eventually they too plateaued. My doctor suggested that I investigate the link between my amalgam fillings and my symptoms.

After much thought and consideration, I met with Dr. Breiner to discuss the possibilities. I decided to have my amalgam fillings replaced. Since I had a mouth full of fillings, two appointments were scheduled to remove and replace them. Within two days of removing the first batch of fillings I slept better, could think more clearly, felt calmer, had more energy and decreased swelling.

Two years after having my mercury laden amalgam fillings removed, I am arthritis free. My weight has returned to 110 pounds. I sleep well every night, have energy, no swelling and no joint pain. Don't try to convince me that mercury in amalgam fillings is harmless. I can't tell you if it was really arthritis or the mercury but I can't argue with these results - can you?

Denise Dolence

CONTENTS

ILLUSTRATIONS

INTRODUCTION

Whatever you do, don't shrug off the concept of "whole -body dentistry" as something to make your teeth healthier. As Dr. Mark Breiner will show you instantly, the art and science of whole-body dentistry is to make your entire body healthier.

To illustrate, as a practitioner of Complementary Medicine, I practice "whole-body medicine", which means I am obliged to look at any and all factors which affect my patients' health. I have found thousands of patients whose health problems were caused wholly or in part by an adverse reaction to generally accepted and widely performed dental procedures.

I have sent many of these patients to Dr. Breiner himself and using the techniques described in this book, he was able not only to pinpoint the cause of my patients' problems, but make a rather accurate estimate of the probability that these patients would benefit from rectifying these dentistry-induced "mistakes."

Rarely were these procedures "mistakes" in regard to preserving the mouth; they proved to be mistakes in preserving the health. So many of my patients overcame serious health problems, such as multiple sclerosis and other auto-immune diseases, that I instruct all my medical staff to take an exhaustive history of every patient's dental procedures.

Just about half my patients give me good reason to question whether or not their illness is caused or contributed to, by silver fillings, mixed fillings, root canals, crowns and other heavy metals known to be toxic to the body.

Dr. Breiner tells the story behind the institution's mismanagement in a matter-of-fact, upbeat tone, a very appropriate accompaniment of the kind of positive information that you'll be reading. But if I were the author, I would paint a picture of criminal negligence and institutional malpractice that is totally unforgivable.

The perpetrators are the American Dental Association, who not only have "stonewalled" the voluminous information about amalgams, but have conducted a relentless witch-hunt in most states to revoke the dentistry licenses of those dentists perceptive, compassionate and courageous enough to allow their patients a safe, viable way to correct these health-compromised procedures.

The ADA has succeeded, not in preserving your health, but in saving their own assets. The impact is that most dentists are convinced that their obviously toxic interventions are completely safe and worth doing repeatedly.

The information this book provides is the only way you can knowledgeably protect yourself against these savage practices.

Robert C. Atkins, M.D.
New York

PART I

DENTISTRY FOR
THE NEW MILLENNIUM

CHAPTER 1

WELCOME
HOW I GOT HERE FROM THERE

In 1972 I was a young army dentist stationed at the White Sands Missile Range in New Mexico. One day my commanding officer, an avid runner, invited me to join him at the track. We began our run together; however, three quarters of the way around the track the effort was too much for me and I could not continue. Winded, exhausted and quite embarrassed, I decided that it was time for me to begin a regular exercise program.

It was an event that would change the entire course of my life. During that year I mounted a determined campaign to improve my physical fitness and began learning about health and nutrition in order to enhance my own well-being.

The more I learned, the more I thought about my dental patients' health. I had always been confused by the fact that some of my patients had extremely healthy oral hygiene habits, yet they would still get tooth decay or gum disease. On the other hand, some of my patients with fairly poor oral hygiene habits would manage to maintain a healthy, cavity-free and disease-free mouth. It just did not make sense.

Slowly I began to apply everything I was learning in my personal quest for better health and nutrition, to my concern about my patients' oral health. I did not change anything in my practice; rather, I shifted my way of thinking and began to notice the relationships between my patients' nutritional habits, their general health, and their teeth.

After leaving the army in 1973, I attended a nutritional seminar led by Dr. Hal Huggins. His approach to nutrition was contrary to much of the conventional wisdom at that time. He also presented information about amalgams (silver fillings) and how the mercury in them may cause adverse health effects. Additionally, the potential danger of adding fluoride to drinking water was discussed. Dr. Huggins seemed like a quack to me. After all, I had learned in dental school that amalgams and fluoride were completely safe and posed no threats whatsoever to human health. I discounted almost everything presented in the seminar without a second thought.

Soon after this, a number of respected dental journals began printing articles about the proper handling of scrap amalgam filling material in dental practices. These articles were advising somewhat stringent precautions to "protect" the dentist and other office staff. Protect us from what, I wondered? Something didn't add up. If mercury was perfectly safe in fillings, then why was the scrap potentially harmful to the dental staff? At the time I made no further investigations into the matter, but the seeds of doubt about mercury had been planted. Five years would pass before I seriously thought about the matter again.

MY TURNING POINT:

In 1978, my dental assistant's five year old daughter, Sarah, had her first cavity. I gladly placed a mercury amalgam filling for her. Two days later she had a seizure. It was a shocking event for Sarah and her family.

Sarah was an active, healthy child who had no history of problems of any kind. She had never had a seizure, and there had never been a disorder of this nature on either side of her family. I remembered instantly that five years earlier, Dr. Huggins had spoken about seizures as a possible effect of mercury amalgam placement.

Even though I found this hard to believe, it was impossible not to consider. Here was a perfectly normal little girl, lively and glowing with energy, struck suddenly - just two days after the filling was inserted.

If the seizure had occurred two months later, probably my suspicions would not have been aroused; however, appearing so soon after the procedure, the coincidence was impossible to ignore. I removed the filling and replaced it with a good-quality composite.

I do not have scientific proof that the filling actually did cause Sarah's seizure. The criteria for "scientific proof" are so stringent that they are virtually impossible to fulfill, working under ordinary clinical conditions. But I do know that this event made me want to find out more about the materials I was placing in my patients' bodies.

I went immediately to the nearest medical library, armed with a lot of questions, to begin my investigation. At this time, I was aware that there was controversy over the safety of amalgam. However, the American Dental Association (ADA) had been adamant all along that it was actually quite safe.

Having faith in the ADA, I was stunned to find an abundance of documented research and scientific data that called into question the safety of amalgam use.

I decided to call the American Dental Association and ask them to send me their information and data relating to this issue. After all, I was a respected, successful dentist, in the prime of my career, and I found this new information hard to reconcile with what I had been taught. I believed the ADA to be a vital professional association. Certainly I did not want to make a rash or erroneous judgement on this issue.

When the ADA materials arrived in the mail, all my illusions about the organization were shattered. Because I had already

Anything we place in the mouth is toxic to some degree, it is a matter of choosing which is least toxic for the patient.

read the scientific studies, I was astounded at the blatant misinformation they were promoting. With all their enormous financial and organizational resources, they did not provide a single valid scientific study to support their position. It was profoundly shocking - and it was a wake-up call for me.

I felt that my patients should be better informed about the possible hazards of mercury amalgam fillings. I started explaining that the material used in their metal fillings consisted of half mercury, and that there were some questions of safety involved. Nearly every patient was upset to learn that mercury was in the amalgam, and did not want it used - even though I could not tell them for sure whether the amalgam might be causing problems. My patients did not think it was worth taking the chance, regardless of whether there was conclusive evidence or not.

Through my research efforts I learned there were a number of symptoms related to mercury poisoning. I started to note which of my patients with amalgam fillings had health problems. I began to mention the idea that maybe their existing health problems could possibly be related to their mercury fillings. Some of them decided to remove the fillings to see what would happen. Interestingly, many of their symptoms significantly improved. I was just as surprised by these results as they were.

During the same time period I had taken a number of courses on the Temporomandibular Joint (TMJ) and similar disorders at the world renowned Pankey Institute for Dentistry. The Institute was teaching dentists about the relationship between bite problems and facial pain, headaches, and TMJ. I began doing bite adjustments for my patients with headaches and facial pain, with excellent results. Interestingly, I noticed that not only were the TMJ symptoms disappearing, but often other symptoms like digestive problems, cold fingers and toes, and endocrine system problems would vanish as well. To make the situation even more intriguing, similar symptoms would also disappear in the patients who had me remove their mercury amalgam fillings.

Clearly there was some common denominator in all these symptoms improving - but I had not been taught about this in dental school. As I became more and more engaged with the positive but inexplicable responses of my patients to various treatments, my research turned a corner. I moved from looking primarily at my patients' mouths and dental procedures as the key to the puzzle, to being fascinated with the body as a whole functioning unit. I began earnestly trying to discover why procedures I would perform in the mouth would effect the rest of my patients' bodies in so strange and profound a manner.

A NEW APPROACH TO DENTISTRY:

In the many years that have passed since these experiences, what I have learned from this quest has completely altered the way I view the body and the way I practice dentistry. I now understand some important principles.

First, all health care practitioners must recognize that *everything we do has implications for our patients*. We must become more aware of these effects and more respectful of the body.

Second, *each patient is unique*. The course and results of treatment must reflect that.

And third, *if you wish to understand the body and healing, you must be willing to explore and learn from new ideas and from your patients' responses*. Just because something has always been done in some certain way does not mean it is right - or that it is right for everyone. Even if our knowledge is very advanced, we must still leave room for growth and new ways of thinking.

Sadly, there are tremendous forces working against new ways

of thinking in the field of dentistry today. Right now an unprecedented number of dentists are being called before state dental boards and are losing their licenses simply because they are removing amalgam fillings. In my opinion, this is occurring because the dental association feels they must protect the position they have held in the past, even when confronted with huge amounts of scientific evidence against such a stance. When one thinks of the silicone implant and asbestos lawsuits, one can only guess at what might happen in the case of dental amalgam.

Unfortunately most dentists rely on the ADA to give them scientific information. Unless they do their own research or actively seek out information about dental amalgam, they will not be aware of the tremendous problems associated with it.

This has prompted the formation of Consumers for Dental Choice, a coalition of citizen groups who have petitioned State Dental Boards, Attorney Generals and governors to stop prosecuting dentists who remove amalgam fillings.

Why are dentists reluctant to change their views? Besides the misinformation from the ADA, I can only guess. For one, it is much easier to practice dentistry when all you have to worry about are the technical aspects of dentistry.

Second, the emotional impact of recognizing that you have been harming people is very powerful and very difficult to deal with. Most dentists choose their profession, at least in part, because of a desire to help other people. It can be devastating to realize that despite all your best intentions, your training and the most stringent attention to your technical skill, you have actually been poisoning your patients - by using a material which you did not know was toxic.

I struggled with this dilemma with a great deal of anguish. Ultimately I resolved it by simply acknowledging that I had done the best that I could with the knowledge I possessed until that point. Now I know that I do not have all the answers, and never will. As we continue to learn more about the materials we use, we may find others that are more toxic than we originally believed. I also know that anything we place in the mouth is toxic to some degree, and it is a matter of choosing which is least toxic for the patient.

I spent five years after I got out of the army studying the technical aspects of dentistry, expending large amounts of time and money, in order to become technically expert. While important, I believe that this is not nearly as critical as the impact of the dental procedures and materials upon the overall health of the patient.

THREE IMPORTANT PRINCIPLES

① Everything we do has implications for our patients.

② Each patient is unique.

③ If you wish to understand the body and healing, you must be willing to explore and learn from new ideas and from your patient's responses.

I never imagined that one day I would be writing this book; I realize that I run great risk in "going public" with this material. However, it is important information, which must be made widely available. Moreover, people have a right to know the implications of dental procedures upon their health.

New information can seem threatening. There is an old adage about how new information is accepted in three distinct stages. The first stage is ridicule; the information is dismissed out of hand. The second stage is vehement opposition and oppression - the phase we find ourselves in now. Ironically, in the third phase, everyone goes around saying, "I always knew that was true." I believe that this book can help accelerate us out of the darkness of oppression and into that final phase of acceptance.

In reading this material, please keep in mind that there are no absolutes in Whole Body Dentistry. The patient's physical, mental and emotional state of being, as well as their lifestyle, must also be examined to understand illness and offer an effective course of treatment. I try not to make blanket recommendations on any specific kinds of procedures. Rather, I am advocating an entirely new paradigm for viewing dentistry in its interactions with the body.

It is my hope that this book will empower people to make informed decisions for themselves and their families, thereby improving their overall health - with all the long-term benefits that such improvement can bring.

CHAPTER 2

A PARADIGM SHIFT

O n the threshold of the twenty-first century, the health sciences in our society are in the midst of a powerful paradigm shift. This is why we see so much friction between the orthodox and alternative medical and dental communities.

The situation has gotten so extreme that in 1991, Congress had to send a directive to the National Institute of Health, demanding that they begin to actively research alternative healing therapies as an option to the "orthodox" methods. A Department of Alternative Medicine was established. According to the AMA Journal, visits to non-traditional healers doubled from 1991 to 1997, with 40% of the population using some form of alternative therapy in 1997. And in 1998, Congress appropriated 50 million dollars for a Center for Complementary and Alternative Medicine within the National Institute of Health.

NEWTONIAN VIEW:

What is the basis of this conflict? Up to now, medicine has been based on a Newtonian view of the world. Man was viewed as a machine, controlled by a computer: the brain and nervous system. This perspective considers man to be a three-dimensional physical body, where the function of the whole can be predicted by the sum of the parts.

> **The ratio of photons to particles of matter is a constant of nature at 9.746 x 10⁸.This ratio means that a science which solely looks at matter is only covering one-billionth of all the phenomena in the cosmos.**
>
> Paraphrase from **Bioresonance and Multi-resonance Therapy,** Vol. 1., Hans Brugeman Ed. Haug Publishers Brussels: English Edition 1993.

Using this simplistic physical map, it follows that treatment will be on a physical plane, using drugs and surgery to effect physical change, whether on the macro or micro molecular level. If the heart malfunctions, give a drug to change its function, or if need be replace it with a new heart or artificial pump. Even if researchers are investigating at a cellular level, they are still observing from the perspective of a cellular, clock-like mechanism. A satisfying aspect of working in this chemical-structural plane is that it is measurable and predictable.

This Newtonian view has led to much advancement in medicine. However, because it is restricted to visible matter, it is extremely self-limiting.

EINSTEINIAN PARADIGM:

As medicine starts to catch up with physics, these limitations will be torn aside. Einstein showed with his famous equation, $E=mc^2$, that energy is matter and matter is energy. In grasping the implications of this, we see that if we are energy, then we in our physical state should also be affected by energy. In this Einsteinian paradigm, we are in fact greater than the sum of our parts, and are multidimensional, composed of many interacting energy fields, with each field having different frequencies. These fields can occupy the same space at the same time, much like the numerous radio, TV and telephone signals that fill the air all around us.

In this model we realize that there is a spark that gives guidance to all this energy. This topic is beautifully discussed in Dr. Deepak Chopra's book, **Quantum Healing**. In that instance between life and death, what is the difference? The person has died, but the cells are still alive. We can still transplant their organs. It is the animating, vital or divine force, which is spiritual and energetic in nature, that is the difference between life and death.

ETHERIC BODY:

Compelling evidence supports the existence of electromagnetic fields which surround each living organism, and which act as a cellular template or blueprint for the physical body. Dr. Richard Gerber, author of the book **Vibrational Medicine,** identifies this field as the "etheric body."[1] This energy field is the software for the development of the body. Without this etheric map, the matter that makes up your body would not know how to organize itself into the body's many organ systems and functions. The etheric body consists of "subtle matter." This is matter which emits a very high, or refined frequency. Physical matter is at a lower or less refined frequency. This high-frequency energy body interacts and communicates with the visible body via energy channels like the acupuncture meridians and the chakras.

ACUPUNCTURE

Biological medical research has discovered that these dynamic human energy systems do indeed have profound impact on the physical body system. Probably most familiar is the work that has been done with the ancient Chinese acupuncture theory. The acupuncture meridian system is a network of energetic pathways that run throughout the body, carrying an invisible energy known as ch'i, which nourishes and vitalizes the organs and tissues of the body. Although there have been many scientific studies documenting the existence of these pathways and the impact of the flow of ch'i energy in the treatment of disease, many Western physicians dismiss the idea.

CHAKRAS

Studies involving EMG electrode readings give evidence that the Indian subtle energy system referred to as the chakras also have a real and measurable impact on the human body. Chakras, generally considered a flaky "new age" idea, are actually energy centers in the body. Each of the seven largest centers corresponds to a nerve plexus and major endocrine gland center. Decreased flow through any one of these energy centers can impact the glands, hormone production, and create all kinds of neural malfunctioning in the physical body.

HOLISTIC APPROACH

Illness in the body will appear as a problem or distortion in the etheric body before it manifests in the physical body. Any injury or sudden disruption to the physical body can be "communicated" to the etheric body in a manner that causes distortion or damage to the etheric body as well. That is why continued study, appreciation, and understanding of the etheric body is essential to developing a holistic approach to getting and staying healthy. You may have heard the term "light body," "emotional body," and "magnetic body" among others. These so-called bodies result from different frequencies being emitted at the subatomic level. Much like different channels on TV, each "program" is broadcast as thousands of pulses of energy of different frequencies, yet each arrives as a complete cohesive picture. The human system also broadcasts several different frequencies of "body," but we have previously been unfamiliar with or unable to perceive most of them. More research is necessary to learn about the multidimensional nature of being human.

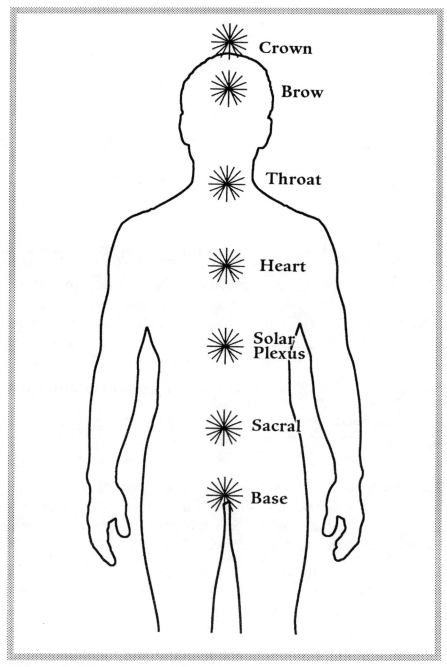

Figure 2.1 Diagram of Chakras

Research has shown that if a leaf is cut, a special type of photograph of this leaf will show the outline (etheric body) of the whole leaf. Also, in any small part of the leaf, there is a hologram of the entire leaf. We thus see that the smallest part of the leaf contains the whole leaf, and from this we can deduce that the smallest part of the universe is a part of the bigger universe, and that it is all connected. This is how plants can communicate with each other, or psychics can see what is happening thousands of miles away.

Illness in the body will appear as a problem or distortion in the etheric body before it manifests in the physical body.

ENERGETIC ASPECTS OF HEALING:

As medicine moves more and more toward the Einsteinian model, treatment and diagnosis beyond the physical become possible. We are beginning to understand through observation and experiments the energetic aspects of healing. From this modern viewpoint, we are slowly coming to a realization how acupuncture, homeopathy, gem stones flower essences, psychic healing, etc. produce their results. They are all interacting with what is called the subtle energy field. Indirectly exploring these fields with EAV or kinesiology *(see respective chapters)* gives insight not otherwise obtainable.

Arriving at an understanding and appreciation of this energetic perspective requires such a shift in thinking, one can understand how those cemented into the Newtonian paradigm would have trouble grasping these new revelations.

However, it is most essential that professionals committed to human health develop the capacity to let go of old, limiting ideas - to constantly transform their thought and practice as new discoveries are made. With a fresh, expanded viewpoint of the human system, the medical community can begin to explore and perhaps say "why not?" to many complementary treatments that were previously dismissed out-of-hand as ridiculous. And once you start experiencing the successful results of some holistic, non-traditional therapies, it becomes impossible to deny their effectiveness.

MY INITIATION INTO ENERGY MEDICINE:

I became aware of the potential of non-traditional therapies after our first son, Adam, had one chronic ear infection after another throughout his infancy. Despite repeated treatment, Adam kept suffering. Antibiotics were given, but soon after they were stopped another ear infection would occur. Finally, after a number of cycles of infections, antibiotics, infections and more antibiotics, the various antibiotics available ceased to be effective.

By the time Adam was three years old, the problems had become so severe that the doctors were concerned that our son might have his hearing permanently impaired. We were told to immediately have tubes placed in his ears. But we knew that the tubes, by allowing drainage, would only stop the symptoms, and would not really cure our son's underlying problem.

We turned to alternative remedies, as many people do, because we were desperate. My wife and I had just started to read about homeopathy, and we decided to try that path before we had our son subjected to general anesthesia and had tubes placed in his ears. Even though I was trained in traditional dental medicine and steeped in the bio-mechanical model of human functioning, Dr.Samuel Hahnemann's original book on homeopathy, **The Organon of Medicine** made a lot of sense to me.

Homeopathy seemed to have a more solid scientific foundation than the modern medical measures I had been taught at dental school. Faced with few options, and terribly concerned about our son, we decided to give Homeopathy a try and found a homeopathic physician. It was a nerve-wracking decision. After all, having a pediatrician, family and friends telling us that we were being foolish and perhaps reckless did not help. Back then (1975), hardly anyone even knew what the word homeopathy meant.

Within a few months Adam's ear problems were cured - and the infections never returned. Homeopathic treatment resulted in a complete reversal of all the symptoms, with resolution of the underlying energetic imbalance. No one was more surprised than I. Homeopathy has been a part of our lives ever since. Not only is my family healthier because of homeopathy, but my patients are also benefitting.

On the threshold of the 21ˢᵗ century, the health sciences in our society are in the midst of a powerful paradigm shift. This is why we see so much friction between the orthodox and alternative medical and dental communities.

We were astonished at the success of homeopathy and also alarmed at how close we had come to allowing the doctors to put tubes in Adam's ears. Over the years, I have referred many children with chronic ear problems to homeopathic physicians (interestingly, many of them were the children of nurses) and all have had their problems resolved.

Even though Dr. Hahnemann uncovered the principles of homeopathy over two hundred years ago, it is based on "modern" energetic principles and emphasizes the mind-body connection. Seeing the results of homeopathy with my son, my consciousness was raised to a new level, and I could no longer ignore the energetic aspects of medicine/dentistry. My odyssey was given new direction.

CHAPTER 3

WHOLE - BODY DENTISTRY™

This year millions of Americans and their children will needlessly suffer a broad range of preventable illnesses. Less serious conditions like excessive fatigue and headaches may go unnoticed or will be incorrectly attributed to aging or stress. Thousands of individuals will develop more serious symptoms like arthritis, colitis, Alzheimer's, heart disease, infections, hypertension, thyroid imbalances, migraines, kidney damage, and even neurological problems. These people will become ill for no apparent reason.

But more often than not, there is a reason for these illnesses: their mouth. The renowned German physician, Dr. Reinhard Voll, based on more than forty years of research and observation, estimated that *nearly 80% of all illness is related entirely or partially to problems in the mouth.* This important statistic would surprise almost all health care practitioners; when I first heard it, it seemed incredible. In fact, both physicians and dentists have been trained to overlook almost entirely the fact that attached to every tooth is a person!

TRADITIONAL APPROACH TO DENTISTRY:

Conventional dentistry takes an extremely limited and mechanistic view of its practice, rarely considering the impact of dental work beyond the frame of the jaw. And there is a disconcerting lack of training on the systemic effects that dental procedures can have on overall body functioning. Dentists have been taught to make treatment decisions without recognizing their impact and with little appreciation of the relationship of the mouth to the rest of the body.

It is critical that patients appreciate the relationship between their mouth and the rest of their body, so they can participate in their own treatment decisions.

Since most dentists have not been trained to look at the entire person as a whole functioning system, they do not recognize the interrelationship of dental procedures and general health. Traditional dentistry has yet to understand how essential the whole-body approach to treatment is to the patient's well-being.

As a result, traditional dental practices can often cause physical illness and trauma, and can actually do more harm than good. The truth is that every dental procedure is an invasion of the human system and may generate an adverse response somewhere in the body. The milder symptoms are often confused with what we have been led to believe are the normal side effects of stress-filled lives, or the natural aging process.

NEW APPROACH TO DENTISTRY:

Seemingly unrelated physical illnesses can be caused by dental problems like non-vital teeth, decay, or impacted wisdom teeth, because of their effect on the body's energetic meridians. In fact, some of the things that we have been told to consider natural or normal may cause completely unnecessary suffering.

That may explain why a new breed of dental practitioner is emerging. These dentists are offering important alternative solutions to traditional dental practices. I like to call this practice "Whole-Body Dentistry."

While, understanding the importance of being a highly skilled and technically proficient practitioner, Whole-Body Dentistry goes beyond this point and takes a broad, holistic view of the dental profession. This all encompassing philosophy recognizes that any work done in the mouth effects the entire human body - often with surprisingly profound results, either positive or negative. By being aware of these relationships, we strive to minimize the invasive quality of these procedures.

Whole-Body Dentistry also interprets information differently. Traditional dentistry has taught us to misread many of the body's cues, because it is still trapped in "old thinking" about the human body. But quantum physics and leading-edge medical theory now indicate that the human system has potential far beyond the prevailing medical model's overly simplistic interpretations.

Consider for a moment that the human body is entirely comprised of billions of tiny particles of energy. Within this energetic system, there are pathways called meridians. Every organ and every part of your body is directly linked to a specific tooth or area of the mouth via these meridians, or energy highways.

This connection is so strong that a Whole-Body Dentist can often accurately "guess" your dental history simply by reviewing your physical symptoms.

For example, a patient came to me with chronic sinus problems which seemed to have no cause or cure. Without even examining him, I immediately asked if he had any root canal work performed on his upper first molar, which relates to the maxillary sinuses. He was amazed that I "guessed" correctly and further conversation uncovered that his sinus problems had indeed begun after the root canal. The offending tooth was removed and within a week his sinusitis completely disappeared.

It can often be that simple. A Whole-Body Dentist is like a detective, sorting through a series of clues and signals and putting the information together in a different way to discover the real source of problems. Often extracting a misaligned or offending tooth will alleviate a whole host of seemingly unrelated physical symptoms in a matter of days. Some problems will actually correct in the chair. I have had patients whose eyesight improved while they were still in the dental chair. You cannot underestimate the impact of your teeth and mouth on your entire body's health.

Getting to know the whole person is an essential first step in eventually making the right treatment decisions. Often dentists do not have the time to get to know their patients personally. However, this is time well spent.

A Whole-Body Dentist must take a detailed medical history, know what kind of work a patient does, and what their lifestyle is like. All of this helps in making a possible diagnosis and in recommending treatment options. It is critical that patients appreciate the relationship between their mouth and the rest of their body, so they can participate in their own treatment decisions. Most patients welcome this information. They feel more in control and less at the mercy of haphazard dental practices which they do not understand.

CHAPTER 4

INTRODUCING YOUR MOUTH

In order to understand **Whole Body Dentistry**, it is important to have a fundamental appreciation for the way the teeth and mouth work, as well as how they interact and function within the context of the rest of the body's processes.

Let us start, then, by describing what your teeth are, how they function and how they are connected to the rest of your body.

If the eyes are the gateways to the soul, then the mouth is the gateway to everything else. It is literally the entrance to your body. Eating, drinking, speaking, smiling and kissing are all functions and pleasures of the mouth. And, of course, your teeth play a vital role in everything your mouth does. For example, what would it be like to try to speak without your teeth? Or eat, or smile, or kiss? Imagine for a moment how Marilyn Monroe would have looked with a missing front tooth, and you will begin to get a picture of how basic our teeth are to self-esteem and the way others view us. That is why most people will go to extreme lengths and money to protect, save and attend to their teeth. Yet very few people actually know the most basic information on the structure of the oral cavity, and how the teeth work.

ANATOMY OF THE TOOTH:

The part of the tooth that you see in your mouth is coated with the familiar white **enamel** which makes the exposed portion of the tooth hard and durable. The hidden part of the tooth is suspended in bone and covered with another material called **cementum**. Ligaments attached to this cementum hold the tooth in place in the bone. These **periodontal ligaments** are somewhat flexible, so that the tooth can move slightly. Sometimes biting on a hard object crushes some of these ligaments and your tooth will be very sore for a few days.

In the center of the tooth is a hollow area, filled with nerve endings, blood and tissue, called the **pulp**. The same blood-filled arteries and networks of nerves that run throughout your body branch off into your mouth, and enter your tooth through the root, running up into the center chamber. Your tooth is literally connected to the rest of your body by the ligaments holding it in place, and also by the blood vessels flowing into it and the nerve endings branching into the root of the tooth. Under the enamel and the cementum is **dentin,** which comprises millions of microscopic tubules.

FLUID FLOW OF TEETH:

We tend to think of teeth as solid, but they are not. The enamel, although quite hard and durable, has tiny tubules running through it which connect to literally millions of other tubules that permeate the dentin. All these tubules are filled with fluid that flows constantly between the dentin and enamel, and through to the nerve endings and blood vessels in the center of the tooth. This fluid provides a constant exchange of nutrients between the tooth and the rest of the body. To show this dynamic interchange, studies have been done in rats. A fluorescent dye was injected into the abdomen of rats and within ten minutes the dye was found in the dentinal tubules.[2]

In a healthy mouth, the fluid flow is from the center out through the tubules into your mouth. In other words, your body delivers nutrients and oxygen through your blood stream into the root of the tooth. The tooth gets "nourished" and passes the fluid out the tubules through the dentin into the enamel.

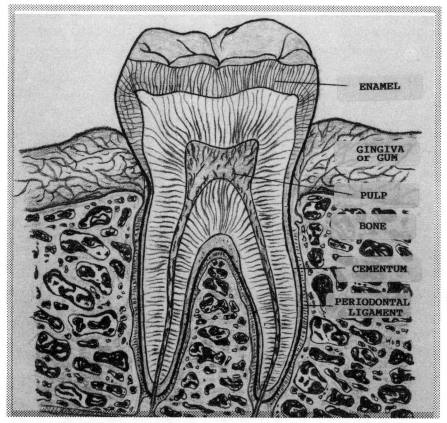

ENAMEL

GINGIVA
or GUM

PULP

BONE

CEMENTUM

PERIODONTAL
LIGAMENT

Figure 4.1 Diagram of tooth

TOOTH DECAY:

This fluid flow is very important in understanding the process of tooth decay. For decay to occur three conditions must be met; (1) you need a specific type of bacteria; (2) you need fermentable carbohydrates; (3) the tooth must be susceptible.

If only the first two are present no decay will take place, or the third can be present, but if you do not have number one or two, no decay will occur. Brushing and flossing help with the first two conditions, but the real key is number three. If the fluid flow is kept in a direction going from the pulp outward decay can be prevented or arrested. This positive outward pressure prevents the penetration of destructive by-products.[3]

If the eyes are the gateways to the soul, then the mouth is the gateway to everything else. Eating, drinking, speaking, smiling and kissing are all functions and pleasures of the mouth.

This fluid flow will be affected by a number of things. Diet is critical - a diet high in refined sugar will cause the flow to go from outward to inward. Stress and lack of certain vitamins and minerals can also do the same thing. I believe that depending on the health of the tissue and organs relating to specific teeth, the fluid flow will be more or less susceptible to change direction. Thus we see, balancing an overall chemistry is a key step in battling the caries (decay) problem. Combine this with proper home care and you have a dynamic duo.

MORE ABOUT TEETH:

The most basic purpose for your teeth is to chew food so you can start the digestive process. The average person has 32 teeth (including the wisdom teeth), in varying shapes and sizes that are suited for specific functions. In your cheeks and under your tongue, you have salivary glands from which digestive enzymes are excreted to help the initial breakdown of food while you are chewing.

If the teeth are not thoroughly cleaned after eating, tiny bits of partially-digested food can cling to the tooth and continue to break down, becoming a feeding ground for bacteria. This causes plaque, which feels like a sticky substance when you run your tongue along your teeth. The bacteria in the deeper part of the plaque now have an anaerobic environment and can produce by-products which could possibly affect the fluid flow in a specific spot on the tooth.

Plaque is easily removed when it is soft. However, if left to harden, it becomes tartar (calculus, in dental language) and must be scraped off during your routine dental cleaning. Tartar can act as a local irritant, much like a pebble in your shoe, causing inflammation in the soft gingival tissues surrounding the tooth.

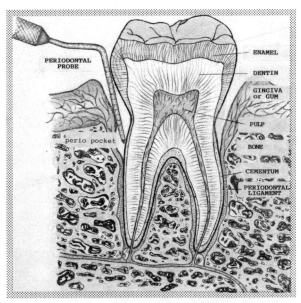

Figure 4.2 Tooth with Periodontal Probe

The **gingival** tissue (gum tissue) surrounds the tooth and provides a covering over the bone in which the tooth is suspended. This gum tissue is like a loose-fitting collar around the tooth, and normally one can measure with a **periodontal probe** one to two millimeters between the tooth and gum.

Some types of disease can cause bone loss, which simply means that the bone shrinks somewhat. In that case the gap between the gum tissue and the teeth can get bigger and create a pocket. The depth of the pocket will now go beyond the normal 1-2 mm often being 6-10 mm. These bacteria-laden pockets and their toxic by-products can further erode the bone and inflame the gum tissue. Tartar can also build up in the pocket. This is how gum disease progresses.

THE LOWER JAW

Your lower jaw bone or **mandible** (*see illustration page 124*) wraps around the bottom of your face and up toward your ears, where it is connected to your skull with a ball and socket joint, called the temporomandibular joint. The socket is in your skull;

the ball, called a **condyle**, forms the top point of the lower jawbone. This joint is cushioned by a **disc** made of cartilage, so the bones do not rub against one another. The condyles are also supported by ligaments; the movement of the jaw is governed by muscles which also connect the mandible to the skull.

In a normal harmonious state, when the lower jaw is at rest, the muscles will also be relaxed and at rest. Sometimes these muscles enter a chronic state of contraction and cause pain. This may lead to TMD or temporomandibular dysfunction. With TMD, the disc which cushions the condyle may be displaced or pushed out of proper position. Pressure or misalignment of the condyle can also impinge upon nerves and blood vessels in the surrounding tissues, and cause a cascade of symptoms, including facial pain, tension headaches, migraines, ringing in the ears, dizziness, stomach problems, toothaches, and much more (*see TMD chapter*).

THE UPPER JAW

The upper jaw, the **maxilla,** where your upper teeth are suspended, is an integral part of the skull. Because the skull bones are large and could be quite heavy, nature wisely hollowed out the bones under your cheeks and behind your nose and forehead. These are your sinus cavities. The upper teeth often rest directly against the sinuses, so any inflammation in the sinus may cause the teeth to hurt. Conversely, problems with the teeth can easily affect the sinuses.

THE TONGUE

An important but often overlooked part of your oral health is the **tongue**. The tongue is a muscle which contains your taste buds, enabling you to taste and enjoy your food. The tongue is far more interesting than most people realize; it offers a great deal of information about a patient's general health and well being. In fact, there are practitioners of oriental medicine who can literally diagnose many illnesses simply by reading the coatings, coloration, indentations, fissures and shape of the tongue.

THE PALATE

By placing your tongue on the roof of your mouth, you can feel the **palate**. The front part is the hard palate; the back is the soft palate. Certain dental appliances may be fitted to rest against the hard palate.

THE TONSILS

Further back in the mouth are the **tonsils** which rest on either side at the entrance to the throat. The health of your tonsils is important, and can be related to your overall dental health. Tonsils are lymph glands and act as filters for toxins from your head.

This overview of the mouth will help in your understanding of the information that follows. Remember, all these "parts" are related to the "whole."

CHAPTER 5

A WHOLE BODY DENTIST'S INITIAL EXAM

A Whole-Body Dentist's initial examination of your mouth should be quite comprehensive. In my own practice, I ask the patient to fill out a detailed health history and sign a sheet which informs them that my views concerning dental amalgams, fluoride and root canals are contrary to those of the American Dental Association.

I then spend some time talking with the patient in a consultation room where we sit face to face. I want to know why they have come to me, what their symptoms are and what they hope to achieve. I also want to know how much research they have done into the area of holistic dentistry.

THE EXAMINATION:

Then we proceed to the examination room. The first exam that I do is a cancer screening and evaluation of throat and tonsil health. In the U.S., 3.6% of all new cancers diagnosed are in the mouth -- some 40,000 new cases of oral cancer are reported yearly. The most frequent sites are the tongue, the floor of the mouth, the gums and the lips.

Next I check to see if the patient has "silver" mercury amalgam fillings, root canals, cavitations (chronic bone infections) or periodontal problems, and whether a misaligned bite could be affecting the mouth adversely. The temporomandibular joint and related muscles for chewing are examined for pain or tenderness. I also check to see if any teeth are loose. I test for hypersensitivity where teeth have been removed, which could indicate that the area never properly healed.

X-RAYS

We also take a panoramic X-ray, which is a screening X-ray of the entire mouth, including the entire jaw bones and sinuses. More detailed X-rays are taken of any suspicious areas. Four "bite-wing" or cavity-detecting X-rays are also taken.

The whole-body approach sometimes leads to a slightly different interpretation of certain symptoms. For example, an area around a root canal done several years ago may appear radiolucent (black) on an X-ray, at which point, traditional interpretation would indicate infection around the roots. But Whole-Body Dentistry recognizes that the so-called "infection" is most likely a positive immunological response by a healthy body to toxins coming from the dead tooth.

SOME IMPORTANT TESTS

As part of the initial visit, the teeth may be checked with electrical instruments to determine their vitality and general health. This process will give insight into whether teeth may be causing symptoms in other parts of the body besides the mouth. Sometimes muscle-testing is used to diagnose problems with teeth. If we can not tell which tooth is causing pain to the patient's upper right jaw, for example, each tooth in the area will be tested kinesiologically to see which one will cause a previously strong muscle to weaken *(see Chapter 22)*. This type of testing has proved to be very accurate. Also, an initial electro-dermal screening is performed *(see Chapter 21)*.

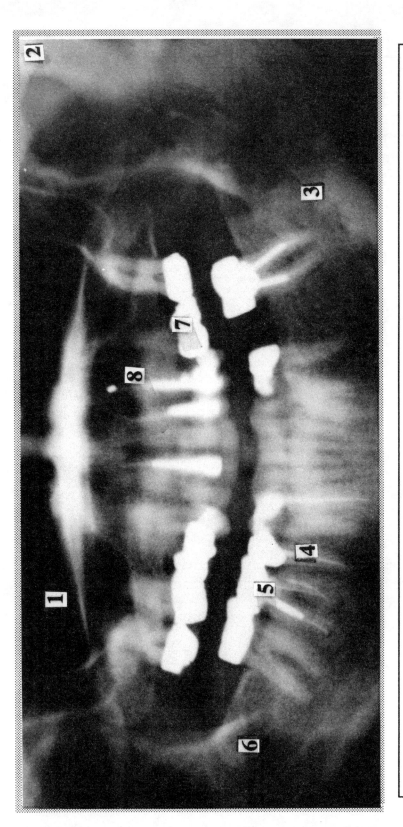

Figure 5.1 Panoramic Dental X-ray

1. Maxillary Sinus
2. Temporomandibular Joint
3. Mandibular nerve
4. Root canal tooth with crown
5. Root canal tooth with crown and post
6. Cavitation
7. Bridge
8. Amalgam placed at root tip after apicoectomy

MERCURY AND ELECTRICITY

It is always important to consider the negative impact metal fillings can have on the patient's health. Eighty-five percent of Americans have at least one cavity filled with "silver" amalgam, which contains large quantities of mercury, a highly toxic metal, more poisonous than arsenic or lead. Most patients improve significantly and some can even completely recover from extremely debilitating diseases, including Multiple Chemical Sensitivity, after having mercury fillings removed.

For most people, removal of mercury fillings is not an automatic cure-all. It can, however, be an essential first step in clearing out the results of toxic and energetic "static" that may be causing a whole host of low-level symptoms. Often accurate medical diagnosis cannot be reached, or treatment will be ineffective, until the symptoms caused by the metals and other problems in the mouth are cleared up.

The electrical charges generated by mercury amalgam fillings are also a threat to your health. The five metals in amalgam fillings (mercury, copper, tin, zinc and silver) when placed in saliva, act as a complete battery generating currents which may interfere with proper cellular function. These electrical currents can cause such seemingly unrelated symptoms such as leg or gastric pain through their impact on the nervous system.

We do not know nearly enough about the effects of these electrical currents; more research is needed. Clinically, high current in the mouth appears to have a negative impact on the entire body, and a direct energetic connection to specific organ or tissue systems can sometimes be observed. Measurement of these currents gives the Whole-Body Dentist more information to help sort out all the pieces involved in the health puzzle.

AFTER THE ORAL EXAM:

After the initial exam, the patient's medical history and report of symptoms are reviewed alongside the results of their oral exam and other test results. I look for energetic links between previous and present problems with the teeth, and whether they relate to the areas of the body which are manifesting symptoms. During this consultation I seek feedback from my patients for additional clues and information. Often blood, urine and trace mineral tests will be ordered at this time.

*R*emoval of mercury fillings is not an automatic cure-all. It can, however, be an essential first step in clearing out the results of toxic and energetic "static" that may be causing a whole host of low-level symptoms. Often accurate medical diagnosis cannot be reached, or treatment will be ineffective, until the symptoms caused by the metals and other problems in the mouth are cleared up.

If it seems there is a clear relationship to their symptoms, and the patient is sure about what they want to do, we may determine a treatment plan at that time. However, if the patient has not done research into the various aspects of Whole Body Dentistry then I prefer that they take the time to do so before coming to a decision.

I usually give my patients reading material. We are then able to discuss the actual treatment plan in great detail on our second meeting. We also review the patient's overall health, lifestyle, and eating habits, as well as anything else that might factor into their ability to heal. Consultations with medical doctors or other appropriate care givers may also be recommended.

In some cases, one or two simple dental procedures will relieve a whole host of problems. In other situations, especially in the case of debilitating diseases, treatment may include removal of mercury fillings, change in diet, and extensive dental work.

At all junctures the patient is always completely aware of the implications of different treatments and makes the final decisions. *The patient is always cognizant that I am not treating their medical problems. I am removing interferences in the mouth that may or may not be related to their symptoms.*

THE PATIENT'S RIGHTS AND RESPONSIBILITIES:

There is a great revolution occurring in the health care industry. Patients are learning to be more actively involved in their own health care and to question the rationale of treatments, their long-term effectiveness, and their potential side effects. Many patients, especially those with chronic or extremely serious illnesses, have gotten tremendous relief from non-traditional and holistic forms of medicine. The one area of medicine that had been neglected in this new wave of health consciousness was dentistry. Now Whole-Body Dentistry is filling that need by presenting a new way of approaching health care.

Whole-Body Dentistry makes a truly radical departure from the way dentistry has been practiced for many years. It can have a powerful effect on your life and health and open new horizons for people who have been termed "chronically ill" or who suffer undiagnosable symptoms.

The Whole-Body approach also raises the issue of integrity and responsibility for the patient's overall health. In recent years, the priorities in making treatment decisions have often become skewed by what is called the "drill, fill and bill" game. Procedures often are selected based on what will be reimbursed by insurance, rather than on the intrinsic value of the procedure. Many patients have relinquished their responsibility for their own health by agreeing with anything as long as it is "covered."

You have a basic right to protect yourself and your family against harmful and invasive procedures which may pose significant health risks. The responsibility for your health care decisions is ultimately yours. What are the possible effects of leaving in an impacted wisdom tooth, or having it removed? What are the pros and cons of root canals, or of having amalgam fillings placed or removed? This book will give you the information that will enable you to understand the basic options, and how different procedures may affect your body and your health.

PART II

DENTAL AMALGAMS

CHAPTER 6

POLITICS AND POISON: METAL IN YOUR MOUTH

When amalgam was first introduced in the United States in 1833, many dentists were outraged at the suggestion of installing such a highly toxic metal in their patients' mouths. In Germany, amalgam was called "Quacksilber" and anyone who placed amalgams was called a "Quack."

This controversy, later termed the First Amalgam War, was quelled when proponents of mercury insisted that the mercury was safe because it was stabilized in the hardened amalgam compound of silver, copper, tin, and zinc, and did not come out. Since amalgam was less expensive and easier to work with than the standard gold fillings, it was not long before silver amalgam was routinely used for filling cavities.

Controversy over amalgam use surfaced again in 1926 and into the 1930's when a German physician, Dr. Alfred Stock, showed that mercury escaped from fillings in the form of a dangerous vapor that could cause significant medical damage. During this Second Amalgam War the American Dental Association vigorously defended silver amalgam and its widespread use was continued. Remarkably, the Food and Drug Administration has separately approved the mercury and the alloy powder for dental use; but the amalgam mixture has never been approved as a dental device. Consequently, in using amalgam, dentists are using a non-FDA-approved device.

The Third Amalgam War began heating up in 1986. Pressure from mounting clinical evidence forced the ADA to finally publicly concede that mercury vapor does escape from the amalgam filling into the patient's mouth. But the ADA remained adamant that mercury in patients' mouths is safe, and in 1986 it changed its code of ethics, making it unethical for a dentist to recommend the removal of amalgam because of mercury. The ADA has actually made it unethical for your dentist to keep you, the consumer, informed of a potential serious health risk, or to recommend a procedure that could possibly improve your emotional and physical health.

"The dentist has a duty to communicate truthfully." ... *the American Dental Association Code of Ethics*

Some dentists have even been accused of unethical behavior and practicing medicine for recommending amalgam removal, in what has become a modern day "witch hunt" against dentists who choose to take into consideration the fact that their patients have poison in their mouths. These fear tactics are being employed by the ADA to make sure that silver amalgam does not come under further scrutiny. This position of this non-scientific dental trade union is most unfortunate.

For years the American Dental Association has insisted that the silver amalgam used for filling cavities is safe. And despite studies showing toxic mercury vapor readings in the mouths of patients with silver amalgam fillings, the American Dental Association still maintains that mercury fillings are safe.

But mercury amalgam is *not* safe. Mercury is unquestionably a toxic substance, and it does indeed escape from amalgam fillings, continuously vaporizing in amounts that are frequently in the hazardous range. Mercury vapor, which is considered the deadliest form of mercury, is inhaled and passes via the lungs into the blood system which carries mercury to virtually all the bodily tissues. It also passes directly into the brain. It is noteworthy that as of October 1998, all over the counter products containing mercury had to be removed from the shelves because the manufacturers could not prove their safety.

VI. From the American Dental Association Principles (Code of Ethics)

Section 3: Principle: Beneficence ("do good")

The dentist has a duty to promote the patient's welfare.

3C. Research and Development

Dentists have the obligation of making the results and benefits of their investigative efforts available to all when they are useful in safeguarding or promoting the health of the public.

Section 5: Principle: Veracity ("truthfulness")

The dentist has a duty to communicate truthfully.

5.A.1. Dental Amalgam

Based on available scientific data the ADA has determined through the adoption of Resolution 42H-1986 (Trans. 1986 .536) that the removal of amalgam restorations from the non-allergic patient for the alleged purpose of removing toxic substances from the body, when such treatment is performed solely at the recommendation or suggestion of the dentist, is improper and unethical.

5.A.2

A dentist who represents that dental treatment recommended or performed by the dentist has the capacity to cure or alleviate diseases, infections or other conditions, when such representations are not based upon accepted scientific knowledge or research, is acting unethically.

5.D.1. Reporting of Adverse Reactions

A dentist who suspects the occurrence of an adverse reaction to a drug or dental device has an obligation to communicate that information to the broader medical and dental community, including, in the case of a serious adverse event, the Food and Drug Administration (FDA).

Figure 6.1 ADA Code of Ethics

VII. From Directions for Use

DENTSPLY CAULK - Dispersalloy^{R} Amalgam

Contraindication

The use of amalgam is contraindicated:

In proximal or occlusal contact to dissimilar metal restorations.

In patients with severe renal deficiency.

In patients with known allergies to amalgam.

For retrograde or endodontic filling.

As a filling material for cast crown.

In children 6 and under.

In expectant mothers.

Side Effects/Warning

Exposure to mercury may cause irritation to skin, eyes, respiratory tract and mucous membrane. In individual cases, hypersensitivity reactions, allergies, or electrochemically caused local reactions have been observed. Due to electrochemical processes, the *lichen planus* of the mucosa may develop.

Mercury may also be a skin sensitizer, pulmonary sensitizer, nephrotoxin and neurotoxin.

After placement or removal of amalgam restorations, there is a temporary increase of the mercury concentration in the blood and urine.

Mercury expressed during condensation and unset amalgam may cause amalgamation or galvanic effect if in contact with other metal restorations. If symptoms persist, the amalgam should be replaced by a different material.

Figure 6.2 Contraindications & warnings from amalgam manufacturer

THE SCIENTIFIC VIEWPOINT:

The scientific evidence for mercury toxicity from amalgam fillings is very compelling. It has been scientifically established:

1. That the mercury in the fillings continuously vaporizes into the mouth air.

2. That this mercury vapor is inhaled and swallowed into the body.

3. That mercury from the fillings is then widely distributed throughout the body, where it stays for very long time periods.

AMALCAP^R PLUS by VIVADENT

Contraindication

Amalcap^R Plus is contraindicated:

- -if proximal or occlusal contacts with other metal restorations are present.
- -if the patient suffers from impaired renal function.
- -if the patient is known to be allergic to amalgam.
- -for retrograde or endodontic restorations
- -as a material for core build-ups under crowns or inlays.
- -for children under six years of age.
- -for pregnant or nursing women.
- -if the stipulated working technique cannot be applied.

Figure 6.3 Contraindications & warnings from amalgam manufacturer

4. That there is a correlation in autopsy studies between amount of mercury in brain tissues and the number, size, and number of surfaces, of amalgam fillings in the mouth.

5. That the mercury absorbed from dental amalgam can cause changes in body chemistry and in organ system functioning - *subtle changes that initially may not be overtly apparent.*

Putting the amount of mercury present in an average filling into perspective, a four-foot fluorescent bulb, which should be disposed of as hazardous waste, has approximately 22 milligrams of mercury. The average dental amalgam filling contains about 1,000 milligrams of mercury.

Some of the most ominous findings related to mercury have been autopsy studies showing that the amount of mercury found in the tissues of the brain directly correlates to the number of mercury amalgam fillings in the mouth.[4]

ALZHEIMER'S DISEASE

These studies take on added significance when one considers the research of Dr. Boyd Haley at the University of Kentucky.

*"**C**hronic, low-level heavy metal poisoning, especially with mercury, is a major health problem that has been virtually unrecognized. As I have been testing for mercury poisoning, I am seeing heavy metal toxicity with increasing frequency, especially in patients with chronic degenerative diseases, chronic fatigue, fibromyalgia, allergies, hypertension, and autoimmune disease. It is crucial to well- being to recognize this health threat."*

Robban Sica, M.D.

Dr. Haley has discovered that patients with Alzheimer's disease have higher than average levels of mercury in the tissues of the brain, establishing a correlation between Alzheimers and mercury amalgam fillings. In one study, Dr. Haley and colleagues exposed rats to levels of mercury vapor comparable to what would be found in people with amalgam fillings. The rats then developed changes in the brain similar to the changes which occur in the brains of Alzheimer patients.[5]

Mercury can travel via various routes from the metal fillings into the rest of the body. The vapor from the fillings can travel through the upper nasal cavity directly into the brain, including the hypothalamus region which regulates heart rate, respiration and blood pressure. It can also travel into the lungs where it can then be absorbed by the blood stream and carried to tissues throughout the body - especially to the kidneys where it accumulates rapidly.

MONKEY AND SHEEP STUDIES

In monkeys, placement of amalgam fillings has impaired kidney function by 60% in sixty days.[6] Fortunately, we have two kidneys and both have a large amount of reserve capacity.

There is also evidence that the mercury in a mother's fillings is passed along to her unborn child. In a very compelling study in Canada by Drs. Fritz Lorscheider and Murray Vimy, amalgam fillings were placed in the teeth of pregnant sheep. The mercury in the fillings was radioactively labeled so that the scientists could definitively trace the mercury to the fillings. Within days, they found the amalgam-related mercury in all the tissues of both the mother sheep and the unborn fetuses, and especially in higher concentrations in the kidneys, thyroid, intestines and jaw bone.[7]

SIDS

A recent German study found that mercury in Sudden Infant Death Syndrome (SIDS) babies brains was directly proportional to the number of fillings in the mother's mouth, providing further compelling evidence that mercury travels to the developing fetus and may be a factor in SIDS.[8]

EFFECTS ON CHILDREN

Many studies on animals and the effects of prenatal exposure to low-level mercury vapor have been done which show adverse effects on brain function. In one test on an isolated group of humans - residents of the Faroe Islands in the Pacific ocean - scientists tested 112 children whose mothers prenatally had hair mercury levels of 10 to 20 mcg per gm (which is considered normal range) compared with controls whose mothers had hair mercury levels of 1 to 2 mcg per gm. At 7 years of age, the former group showed mild decrements relative to controls in motor function, language and memory.[9] Is this why the manufacturers of dental amalgam caution against placement of dental amalgam in pregnant women?

EFFECTS ON BLOOD VALUES

A study that has not yet been published as of this writing, which was funded by the Coors Foundation, is very enlightening. Researchers took healthy subjects who had from three to ten amalgams. They had no root canals or other metals in their mouths. Blood testing was done to check, among other things, white blood cell counts - to reflect immune system functioning; oxyhemoglobin levels; cholesterol values; and a whole host of other parameters. They then removed the amalgams, replaced them with composites, and took a second set of blood samples. The removal of the amalgams affected the numbers in a positive direction. The white blood cell counts settle into a narrow corridor of 5-6,000. Venous oxyhemoglobin, which measures the actual percentage of oxygen saturation, increased in twenty out of twenty-seven patients. Low cholesterol values went up and high values came down toward the optimal two hundred and twenty-two. The composites were

were then removed and the amalgams reinserted. The blood results were affected in a negative manner. A second removal of the amalgams again caused a positive change in blood test results.[10]

CLINICAL EVIDENCE:

Many dentists are rapidly discovering that their patients are recovering from a broad range of illnesses when their silver amalgam fillings are replaced with less toxic materials. *(see Chart of Symptoms at end of chapter)* People who were barely functioning have regained all or most of their faculties. Sometimes the recoveries are fairly rapid. There are thousands of anecdotal reports by dentists, allergists and other medical professionals attesting to the link between becoming "mercury free" and a fast, dramatic, and otherwise inexplicable improvement in symptoms.

There are many more cases unreported in which the improvement is being termed spontaneous remission. At this point many doctors refuse to believe in any link between amalgam fillings and ill health, even when the positive results of removing those fillings are staring them right in the face.

The ADA calls the mounting anecdotal evidence insignificant and argues that there is no proof that mercury fillings are unsafe. But many of the recoveries are so immediate, so dramatic, that you would hardly need to be a trained clinician to make the obvious assumption.

You have to begin to wonder: why are we arguing over whether a poison is a poison?

One reason may be that it is particularly difficult to pinpoint the symptoms of mercury poisoning. Mercury poisoning is nothing new; in fact, the expression "mad as a hatter" refers to mercury poisoning contracted by hatters, who processed hat felt using mercuric chloride. The hatters would often develop mental illness

DENTAL DETECTIVE STORY

DEPRESSION

Soon after 60 Minutes aired its exposé on mercury amalgam on December 16, 1990, Melanie came to my office. She suffered from severe depression which had greatly worsened after breaking a tooth which exposed a new surface of amalgam. She wanted to have all her amalgams removed immediately. Melanie was under psychiatric care which was not helping; her psychiatrist supported her wish to see if amalgam removal could make a difference. She told me that she was feeling suicidal and out of control, and did not want to wait to have the procedure done.

We gave her some vitamins, minerals and homeopathics to prepare her for the removal and set up an appointment for the removal several days later.

Melanie's reaction to the mercury removal was dramatic. Her depression lifted soon thereafter and she rapidly became a normal, healthy woman. Melanie feels absolutely certain that she would have killed herself if the mercury had not been removed. So certain, in fact, that she sent a letter to Morley Safer, thanking him and 60 Minutes for helping to save her life.

as a result of their high exposure to mercury.

The symptoms associated with low level mercury poisoning (micromercurialism) range across a very broad spectrum. Some of the effects of low level exposure are commonly attributed to stress or aging, like inexplicable fatigue, loss of memory or inability to concentrate, moodiness, anxiety, lack of confidence and even severe depression.

A great deal is known medically about acute reactions to high levels of exposure, but very little is known about the kind of low-level daily exposure caused by mercury fillings called micromercurialism. One person may simply feel tired and get mild chronic headaches; another may develop arthritis, migraines or acute colitis, while yet another may become completely debilitated by Multiple Sclerosis like symptoms.[11]

Y ou have to begin to wonder: why are we arguing over whether a poison is a poison?

I feel that heavy metal toxicity from exposure to small amounts of the toxin is the most overlooked problem in medicine and dentistry today. Diagnosis is very difficult to make, if one is not trained to look for this link.

A recent study of 34 practicing dentists and 15 dental assistants has shown adverse effects of cumulative low-level mercury exposure. All had very low urinary mercury levels, and had "alteration in moods, deficits in motor function, and subtle losses in memory and visuo-spatial cognitive skills" that were shown to be related to mercury body burden. Most significant was the fact that the subject's urinary mercury levels are comparable to the general U.S. population, raising questions as to the effects of amalgam.[12]

This broad range of systemic response to mercury is based on an individual's threshold and resistance to toxicity. Many people have what is termed a "high threshold" for toxicity. They may have had mercury fillings for years without experiencing any overt problems. Other persons exposed to the exact same levels of mercury may have dramatically different reactions and symptoms.

But even people who seemingly have a high tolerance to amalgam need to be aware of the impact mercury and alien electrical impulses have on the human body. Many of the symptoms that are unfortunately considered "normal," such as headaches, stomach troubles, sinus problems and many other discomforts, may be related to the metals in your mouth.

In the case of serious illness, removal of mercury amalgam fillings often clears up a whole host of low intensity symptoms which literally interfere with an accurate medical diagnosis. Amalgam removal could very well become the single most important step in enabling your physician to help you get well. Often an accurate medical diagnosis cannot be reached until the problems in the mouth are cleared. The effect of mercury is like static on the radio: it interferes with the diagnostic process. You cannot really get a clear signal until the static is removed.

As a consumer you have a right to know the danger to you and your children of having mercury fillings. Last year, more than 100 million silver amalgam fillings containing 50%, or about one gram (1000 milligrams) of mercury per filling were placed in patients' mouths. If you have these poisonous fillings, then you are inhaling toxic mercury vapor every day.

I have only briefly touched upon the effects and research with reference to amalgam. See the recommended reading list for more books that deal in depth with the mercury issue.

I believe we will look back one day and recognize that mercury amalgam significantly contributed to many of our "modern" illnesses and symptoms. In the second part of this book I discuss the actual process of mercury removal in greater detail. If you have amalgam fillings, I urge you to review that section and then find a good Whole-Body Dentist who can discuss how your body may be reacting to the exposure and what courses of action are available.

In concluding this chapter let me ask this: Why is the mercury before it goes into the mouth a hazardous toxin, and why does the scrap amalgam, which is removed from the mouth, have to be stored in a special manner and taken away by a licensed hazardous waste company? If you ignore all the science and just use common sense, you realize how absurd the position of the pro amalgamists is. It seems they believe that the only safe place to store mercury is in the mouth!

ELEMENTAL MERCURY VAPOR EXPOSURE
1. PSYCHOLOGICAL DISTURBANCES (Erethism):

Irritability
Nervousness
Shyness or timidity
Loss of memory
Lack of attention
Loss of self-confidence
Decline of intellect
Lack of self-control
Fits of anger
Depression
Anxiety
Drowsiness
Insomnia

2. ORAL CAVITY DISORDERS:

Bleeding gums
Alveolar bone loss
Loosening of teeth
Excessive salivation
Foul breath
Metallic taste
Leukoplakia   (white patches)
Gingivitis (inflammation of the gums)
Stomatitis (mouth inflammation)
Ulceration of gingiva, palate, tongue
Burning sensation in mouth or throat
Tissue pigmentation

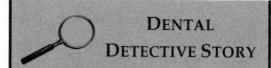

DENTAL DETECTIVE STORY

PSYCHOLOGICAL DISTURBANCES

Serena, referred by a psychiatrist, had many emotional problems. Among them was a fear of letting anyone get close to her physically. She did not like the idea of dental treatment because of the close proximity of me and my assistant during dental procedures. She was also very shy and nervous. Her PMS was so bad, she had tried to commit suicide several times. A few months after amalgam removal it was very gratifying to have her come in and give me a warm hug of thanks.

3. GASTROINTESTINAL EFFECTS:

Abdominal cramps
Constipation or diarrhea
Gastrointestinal problems
   including colitis

4. SYSTEMIC EFFECTS:

CARDIOVASCULAR:
Irregular heartbeat
   (tachycardia, bradycardia)
Feeble and irregular pulse
Alterations in blood pressure
Pain or pressure in chest

NEUROLOGICAL:
Chronic or frequent
   headaches
Dizziness
Ringing or noises in ears
   Fine tremors (hands, feet,
   lips, eyelids, tongue)

RESPIRATORY:
Persistent cough
Emphysema
Shallow and irregular
   respiration

IMMUNOLOGICAL:
Allergies
Asthma
Rhinitis (inflammation of the nose)
Sinusitis
Lymphadenopathy, especially cervical (neck)

DENTAL DETECTIVE STORY:
IMMUNOLOGICAL DISORDERS

Louis was a 47-year old salesman who sounded like he had a terrible cold. His sinuses were so blocked that he had a nasal sound which made him very self conscious. He felt this was adversely affecting his career. Louis was told that surgery to remove polyps in his nose might help. He also was very distraught because he could no longer sing in his barber shop quartet. Another problem was that he had asthma attacks with each meal. A few months after amalgam removal his ENT doctor inquired as to who did his surgery - the polyps were gone. His asthma attacks were also gone and Louis was back singing.

ENDOCRINE:

Subnormal temperature
Cold, clammy skin,
    especially hands and feet
Excessive perspiration

OTHER:

Muscle weakness
Speech disorders
Dim or double vision
Fatigue
Anemia
Hypoxia (lack of oxygen)
Edema (swelling)
Loss of appetite (anorexia)
Loss of weight
Joint pains

5. SEVERE CASES:

Hallucinations
Manic depression

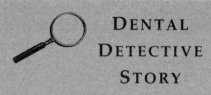

DENTAL DETECTIVE STORY

FATIGUE

Sally was a 38-year-old who suffered from Chronic Fatigue Syndrome. She was unable to work because she would be in bed for a large part of the day. She had tried many forms of treatment and was taking numerous supplements. Naturally, she was very depressed about the whole situation. Previous to her getting ill, she was able to work, take care of her two children, and manage her household.

Having read about the effects of mercury inhibiting the binding of oxygen to hemoglobin, thus improving energy, she wanted her fillings out. Shortly after removal, she had to be cautioned to slow down. Sally said she had a lot of "catching up to do."

Chart of Symptoms of Mercury Toxicity reprinted with permission from BioProbe, Inc.

ORGANIC MERCURY EXPOSURE*
(chart reprinted from Bio-Probe, Inc.)

1. EARLIEST SYMPTOMS:

Fatigue
Headache
Forgetfulness
Inability to concentrate
Apathy
Depression
Outbursts of anger
Decline of intellect

2. LATER FINDINGS:

Numbness and tingling of
    hands, feet, lips
Muscle weakness progressing
    to paralysis
Dim or restricted vision
Hearing difficulty
Speech disorders
Loss of memory
Incoordination
Emotional instability
Dermatitis
Renal damage (kidney)
General central nervous
    system dysfunction

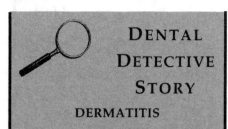

DENTAL DETECTIVE STORY

DERMATITIS

Tony was 28 years old and embarrassed by the rash on his arms and legs. The rash was bright red with lots of pimples. He was particularly unhappy in the summer, when short sleeved shirts and bathing suits were needed. Tony had tried several types of diets and supplement regimens without the hoped for result. Cortisone creams helped but he used them only with the worst flare-ups. He was afraid of the possible side effects from long term cortisone use.

A friend told him to have his mercury fillings removed; it seemed her acne had been helped by this. Removal of the fillings brought Tony the clear skin he had sought.

(Mouth bacteria have been shown to convert some of the mercury released by amalgam fillings into organic mercury)

CHAPTER 7

ELECTRICAL PROBLEMS

I would estimate that about half of the problems I see in my patients are related to electrical currents caused by dissimilar metals in the mouth. Any chemical engineer can tell you that when you put two different metals together in a salt solution, similar to saliva, electrical current is generated. Essentially the metals act as a battery, and depending upon which metals you combine, the amount of electricity generated can vary.

The amount of electricity generated would seem quite small, until you consider that your entire nervous system is managed by a very small electrical current. In fact, the five metals in amalgam, when placed in saliva, could generate enough current to interfere with your brain or heart function. When you begin to understand the impact of even a subtle electrical charge on your nervous system, it is actually surprising that this link has remained so elusive. Every action you take, every thought you have is propelled into bodily function by tiny electrical impulses jumping across the synapses in your nervous system and across cell membranes. These electrical messages are actually a form of language that the nervous system decodes and relays, for example, from your brain to your hand. Some of these are conscious, like when you decide to turn the pages of this book.

Every hour billions of electrical impulses create an automatic messaging system that keeps your body functioning as a highly sophisticated series of processes. Everything from the production of blood cells to the rate at which your bones deteriorate is controlled by the network of electrical impulses in the nervous system. The electrical "messages" emanating from the metals in your mouth may be in disharmony and interfere with your normal electrical signals. It should hardly seem remarkable that this current could make you ill.

To evaluate the electrical impact of metals on my patients, I use a device called a Pertec instrument which measures electricity in three ways: the voltage or potential energy; the amperage or current, which is the actual flow of electrons; and the milliwatt per seconds, which is the amount of force behind the flow.

Studies from Europe indicate that it is considered acceptable for teeth to emit electricity below 100 millivolts and three micro amps. In Linda, the patient in the Dental Detective Story in this chapter, I measured a whopping 980 millivolts in one upper molar!

Many of my patients' fillings exceed the norms, especially when gold or other metals are in the mouth along with amalgams.

***W**hen a problem clears up instantaneously or within a few hours, then I can logically assume it was electrical in nature. Mercury does not leave the body this quickly.*

In my experience, excess current floating around your body can have a very serious impact. Because the current flows through the path of least resistance, it is very difficult to predict the effects, or where the resulting problems will occur. Diagnosing the impact is difficult, and a lot of research is needed in this area.

Interestingly, more than 50 years ago, the ADA Journal included studies about the systemic effects of these galvanic currents.[13] The article noted the symptoms of galvanism as being:

1. Metallic or salty taste.

2. Increased salivary secretion.

3. Burning or tingling sensation along the tongue.

4. Occasional nerve shocks and pulp sensitivity from connecting restorations or by connections made with a spoon or fork.

5. Pathological changes in the blood, kidney or organs, probably caused by absorption of ionized toxic metals.

6. Generalized discomfort in the mouth, irritability, indigestion, loss of weight, and in some cases, reflex radiating neurologic pains through branches of the fifth trigeminal nerve.

When I see a problem clear up instantaneously or within a few hours, then I can logically assume it was electrical in nature. Mercury does not leave the body this quickly. At least half of the improvements reported to me by my patients fall into this category. When 60 Minutes did their show in 1990 about amalgams, one of the people interviewed described how she got out of her wheelchair in a few hours. The ADA said this could not have happened so quickly if she had been mercury toxic. I agree; I think it was in fact an electrical response.

CHAPTER 8

MERCURY AMALGAM REMOVAL

In December 1990, the award winning television news program, 60 Minutes, aired a story called "Is There Poison in Your Mouth?" which focused on the controversy over mercury amalgam fillings. The viewing public responded in droves requesting dentists across the country to remove their amalgam fillings. Many dentists reacted to this pressure and replaced their patients' fillings even though they were not adequately trained to do so.

PRECAUTIONS:

I received literally hundreds of calls during the months following that broadcast from patients who had their fillings removed and then became very ill. Why? Because mercury is a deadly poison and an oxidant catalyst, and removing more than one filling from people who are already ill, or are unknowingly near their toxic threshold, can make the individual worse unless correct safety precautions are used.

These safety precautions not only encompass such things as having the patient breathe oxygen during removal, using large amounts of water, intravenous Vitamin C, etc. - but more importantly addressing the patient's level of toxicity and body chemistry before ever starting.

Amalgam fillings should never be removed without adequate testing. First, your dentist needs to evaluate how your body is currently handling the poison it has already absorbed. Are your tissues so blocked with toxins that you cannot excrete mercury adequately? Are your kidneys strong enough to handle the extra burden? The use of hair and blood analysis and a detailed symptom history is extremely valuable at this point. Cooperation with the patient's physician or complementary health care provider is also helpful. Some supplementation with vitamins, minerals and homeopathics is necessary to help balance the chemistry, to facilitate excretion, and to protect against the increased exposure resulting from removal and the ensuing dumping of mercury.

When it comes to amalgam removal, we have to consider the results of toxic accumulation. Often you can point to a direct effect. I believe that in most cases it is wise to remove toxic metals from the mouth. Moreover, it is usually true that by the time a patient gets to me, they are already seriously ill or plagued with confusing symptoms for which no one can seem to find a diagnosis or solution. In these cases, almost all patients request that I remove their amalgam fillings, even though they have no firm assurance that their health problems will be alleviated.

TESTING:

For an otherwise healthy patient, the decision whether to remove or not remove their amalgams is related to how preventive they want to be. If patients want to consider the impact mercury may be having on their health, many tests can be used. A provocative urine test can reveal how much saturation of mercury is in the tissues of the body. We begin by having a physician take a baseline urine test for mercury and other heavy metals. Then a chelating drug which binds the metals is administered. When the urine is retested, you can see if there is a substantial increase of metals in the urine, compared to the baseline, indicating a problem with a metal buildup in the tissues.

Some dentists use a mercury vapor test which helps determine how much mercury vapor is escaping the fillings both during stimulation (like chewing) and while at rest. A dental materials compatibility test will tell immunologically if you are reacting to components in the mercury filling *(see Chapter 9)*. I also use Electro-Dermal testing to help evaluate the impact of the mercury fillings on the body's meridians.

*F**or an otherwise healthy patient, the decision whether to remove or not remove their amalgams is related to how preventive they want to be.***

CLUES TO TOXICITY:

It is important to take a thorough patient health history. Often a clear connection between the onset of symptoms and amalgam placement can be established. Another clue that I have found useful has to do with thyroid patients. I spent a few days with Dr. Broda Barnes, author (with Lawrence Galton) of **HYPOTHYROIDISM: The Unsuspected Illness**. Dr. Barnes would administer thyroid medication on the basis of a low basal body temperature. I found it interesting that often the basal temperature would not increase, necessitating more and more thyroid medication over time. Over the years it has been my experience that when the basal temperature does not increase upon taking thyroid medication, it is because of an underlying heavy-metal problem, usually mercury.

There are a few other clues that usually indicate a system blocked with mercury. Candidiasis is an overgrowth of a normally occurring gastrointestinal fungus. When mercury is present, it can upset the normal balance of flora in the gut and allow the Candida albicans fungus to get out of control. When a patient tells me that they have a candida problem that cannot be cured or that keeps reoccurring, you can bet that they have a heavy metal problem.

When a patient relates that they go for chiropractic adjustments and their neck or some other vertebrae can never "hold" the adjustment, the problem is usually in the mouth. Often it will be due to mercury toxicity from the amalgams or the electrical component from the amalgams. However, the connection is not as clear as with the thyroid or Candida symptoms because root canals, wisdom teeth or the bite can also cause a weakness in the vertebral area.

*R*emoving more than one filling from people who are already ill, or are unknowingly near their toxic threshold, can make the individual worse unless correct safety precautions are used.

BEFORE ACTUAL REMOVAL:

When the decision is reached to remove the fillings, we want to ensure that the body is working efficiently and regularly. The bowel is the major excretory route for mercury, so it is essential that a patient's elimination system be functioning properly before we begin the process of removal. Once the constant low-level source of mercury is removed, the body begins a process of detoxification; the mercury that is released must be able to leave the body rapidly and completely. Part of the pre-removal preparation might include vitamins, minerals and other supplements as well as homeopathic remedies.

I will usually place my patients on some herbs or homeopathics to help support the liver and/or kidneys. Solidago is a good kidney herb and silymarin is excellent for the liver. Based on EAV, blood and/or hair analysis, supplementation will be given prior to amalgam removal. I tend to use food derived supplements (*see chapter 25*). However, there are certain fractionated vitamins and minerals that have been shown in the scientific literature to be beneficial to the mercury toxic patient.

The following is a list of some of these supplements with recommended dosages:[14]

1. glutathione   50 milligrams three times per day

2. N-acetyl-L-Cysteine (NAC) 250mg two times per day

3. Methionine   1000 milligrams per day divided into two or three doses.

4. Vitamin B_6 50 milligrams per day

5. Vitamin C   500 milligrams three times per day

6. Zinc   15-30 milligrams per day

7. Magnesium   200 milligrams per day

8. Selenium   50 micrograms per day

9. Garlic

It is best to let whoever is "quarter backing" your removal regimen, decide what your supplementation program should consist of.

REMOVAL APPOINTMENT:

The body's immune system runs on a seven-day cycle. This means that seven days after amalgam removal, the immune system will not be able to tolerate another insult from removal as well as on, i.e., the fourth or the ninth day. Appointments are thus scheduled accordingly.

During the removal my assistant and I wear mercury vapor masks to protect ourselves. The average dentist has a thousand times more mercury in his or her pituitary gland than the average person. Several precautions are necessary for the patient, including a nose mask for breathing oxygen, a rubber dam to cover the patient's mouth, a lot of water coming from the drill, and special high speed suction. To decrease the amount of vapor, we section the fillings out in chunks as opposed to grinding it out. I use an electric drill for two reasons. First, because it cuts so much more efficiently than an air turbine, I can chunk out the amalgam faster. Second, because it turns at slower revolutions per minute, there is less chance of heating the tooth, thereby creating pulpal damage. Consequently, it is rare that a patient has a tooth die after mercury removal.

We also use air filters for the treatment room where the removal takes place. Intravenous vitamin C is administered because its antioxidant effects help to minimize the impact of mercury entering the bloodstream. Generally it is best to get all the mercury out as quickly as possible; over the years I have found that the longer the process is, the more stressful it is for the patient both mentally and physically.

Mercury loves sulphur and eagerly bonds with it. Because sulfur is so prevalent throughout our bodies this is a primary way in which mercury interferes with proper functioning. Therefore, I ask my mercury-removal patients to include eggs in their diet because eggs have a high sulphur content. The mercury binds with the sulphur from the eggs and takes it out of the system.

Diet and nutrition factor heavily in a patient's ability to process the toxins out of the system (see chapter 9). Detoxifying baths, sauna and exercise are important because they help the patient literally "sweat out" the poisons. I may also advise my patients to receive massage, acupuncture, homeopathy or regular medical treatment to assist in the healing process.

CHAPTER 9

DETOXIFICATION AFTER MERCURY AMALGAM REMOVAL

(Written in conjunction with Warren M. Levin, M.D.)

A malgam fillings are the major source of mercury burden in the average person. Thus it seems apparent that amalgam removal is the necessary first step in helping a patient who is mercury-toxic.

However, according to Warren Levin, M.D., who was one of the first physicians in the country to treat mercury-toxic patients, medical, social or economic factors may combine to make this ideal protocol impossible. It is probable that some detoxification of the body can be accomplished temporarily without replacing all the fillings. However, this will not be effective in patients with an allergy to mercury, or with symptoms caused by electricity in the mouth.

Dr. Levin notes that he has tested many patients - he was his own first subject - who had all their amalgams removed more than ten years previously. **All of these patients, including Dr. Levin himself, were still burdened with residual mercury contamination of the body.** Thus, removing the mercury from the mouth is getting rid of the primary source of mercury, but it is not the end of the process. The mercury must then be removed from the tissues and organs. To accomplish this, the body usually needs some assistance.

SUPPORT:

There are many things that can help. First, Dr. Levin says it is essential that the patient continue on a proper nutritional program and any supplements that have been found necessary. In general, high levels of sulfur-containing foods, such as egg yolks, and supplements, such as glutathione and selenium, are critically important because these binding agents are constantly lost in urine, bowel movements and sweat, and must be replenished on a daily basis.

Usually before removal, patients are already taking specific detoxifiers recommended by their physicians. I often find giving three specific Hoban homeopathic combination products beneficial. One is for support of the organs in general, especially the liver and kidneys. Another is specific for helping to pull dental metals out of the tissues, and the third is to help them exit from the body.

Sometimes before amalgam removal, but almost always after, I will have the patients take the herbal concentrate Cilantro. This helps release mercury from the tissues. Chlorella is also recommended to help mercury excretion. If the Hoban homeopathic products are not being used, it is very important to support the kidneys and/or the liver with herbs or homeopathics.

EXCRETORY ROUTES:

The skin is a huge excretory organ and anything that helps a patient sweat is useful. A word of caution, however; metallic toxins accumulate in fat, and mobilizing the toxins from fat too quickly can be counterproductive, especially if chelators are not used. Any type of stress factor will mobilize fatty deposits to meet metabolic needs. Besides sweating, any kind of physical or emotional stress, including illness or fasting - even the normal overnight fast during sleep - can release toxins from fat as well.

Therefore, depending upon the individual, exercise or saunas may not be a good idea in the initial phase of detoxification.

Detoxification baths are excellent, and formulas for these are in the appendix. Various forms of massage therapy that help the lymphatic drainage system can also be very helpful. A rebounder is also an excellent lymphatic stimulator.

Feces are the major route of mercury excretion, followed by the urine. As stated before, it is essential to have proper daily elimination. Because the health of the colon is so important in anyone trying to improve their well-being, many people find colonics to be of great benefit. Vitamin C in megadoses with magnesium will usually increase fecal elimination. (Check this protocol with your health care practitioner).

As a person is working on removing their mercury burden, their status is very easily monitored with the Umbilicus Test. (*See Chapter 22*).

DMPS:

If progress is not proceeding rapidly enough or a roadblock is reached, the physician will usually recommend giving DMPS intravenously. DMPS (2,3 dimercapto-1-propane sulfonic acid) is a very powerful chelator of mercury. It has been used in Russia, Germany, Japan and Sweden for more than 25 years as the treatment of choice for mercury poisoning. DMPS is administered when doing a provoked urine test when originally testing for mercury burden. Beneficially DMPS will also chelate lead, tin, aluminum, copper, and other heavy metals. Concurrent with DMPS administration, because some essential minerals are also chelated out, the physician will give intravenous mineral replacement the day after DMPS is given, or will prescribe specific minerals to be taken orally.

Dr. Levin is part of a nationwide study of the effectiveness of DMPS and of this regimen in detoxifying mercury-toxic patients. Although the study will not conclude for several years, Dr. Levin notes that he has seen remarkable results among his own patient population using the study protocol.

*R*emoving mercury from the mouth is getting rid of the primary source - but it is not the end of the process. The mercury must then be removed from the tissues and organs.

Physicians knowledgeable in metal toxicity may also use DMSA (2,3 dimercaptosuccinic acid) which is given in an oral form marketed as Chemet, or as the pure material from a "compounding" pharmacy. Dr. Levin notes that there is a concern as of this writing that DMSA, which crosses the blood-brain barrier, may be contraindicated in patients with a high body burden of mercury because it might carry mercury *into* the central nervous system, whereas DMPS will not do this. Therefore Dr. Levin says that DMPS is used first until the excretion is low (less than three mcg/24 hours.) At that point DMSA may be given with excellent safety.

OTHER FACTORS:

When a patient's metal burden is lowered, and they are still suffering from a number of ailments, the physician and I immediately think about root canals and cavitations, both of which can cause significant system malfunctions. The best means of isolating these problems is with EAV or kinesiology, because they can energetically determine if the problems are still being caused by something in the mouth.

PART III

DENTISTRY
AND
YOUR HEALTH

CHAPTER 10

COMPATIBILITY TESTING
FOR
DENTAL MATERIALS

The materials used in dental work must be strong enough to do the job. That is why most dentists use alloys or combinations of metals which may include copper, palladium, platinum, silver, and others. However, there are now alternative materials which are preferable and more than adequate to accomplish the task.

If possible, always avoid metal in the mouth and opt for a porcelain based or ceramic composite material. This warning is especially important if there is already amalgam present. The presence of other metals will cause increased electrical currents, and therefore greater corrosion of the amalgam. This results in even higher levels of toxic by-products being released into the body.

If you are ill, never proceed with any dental work until you have had a compatibility test. This test, also called a Dental Materials Reactivity Test, is performed by a special laboratory to determine which materials your system will be least sensitive to. The test considers metals as well as composites, cements, and other dental components which can often cause immunological reactions.

Blood is drawn, and the serum which contains the white cells - and hence the person's antibodies - are separated. Antibodies are those complexes formed in response to something foreign when the first line of defense has been breached and a more systemic response is required. Placing the serum in a small well which contains a minute amount of a dental material component, i.e., silver, will cause an agglutination reaction or no reaction. A reaction indicates that antibodies to the material are present. This means the person's immune system has been sensitized to the particular material and any further encounter with that material may lead to autoimmune reactions or a whole host of reaction symptoms, as seen with mercury toxicity. The challenge of serum against over 150 components of dental materials is done. All positive responses are fed into a computer, and cross-checked against the ingredients in most brand-name products. The ensuing printout will indicate by manufacturer's name what materials are immunologically reactive and are to be avoided, as well as those which may be used. Even if one were to use a material deemed not suitable, because no visible reaction had occurred with its use in the mouth prior to the compatibility test, it is still inappropriate treatment.

Because of differences in compensation, tolerance, and dose and time factors, one cannot know when an individual's threshold is being approached. Consequently, in a perfect world, everyone should have a compatibility test.

AMALGAM SUBSTITUTES:

Naturally we need to replace the amalgam fillings we have removed. There are choices as to which alternative materials to use. Bear in mind that any foreign material in the mouth can be considered "toxic" and may have a resultant negative impact. However, when compared to mercury, many of the available nonmetallic materials appear relatively benign. We can also minimize the impact by testing the materials for biological compatibility with the individual patient, so the least offensive material can be used.

Ordinarily I use a plastic/glass composite tooth-colored material. The composite filling is a material which does not weaken the teeth like amalgam fillings. Since they are white, they are also far more attractive than a mouth full of gray metal. Studies indicate that because composites are a long-chain polymer, they are not readily absorbed and are therefore fairly bio-compatible - if immunological testing has determined that particular composite to be appropriate for that individual.

Patients are often concerned about the process of bonding the filling to the teeth, and what kinds of problems could occur. Surprisingly enough, the bonding process by which the filling is adhering to the tooth actually strengthens the tooth. Some teeth containing bonded composites are almost as strong as a virgin tooth. Composite materials are, however, very technique-sensitive, which means that the dentist must be skilled and meticulous in using these materials. I have heard of many cases of composite bonded fillings failing, allowing leakage and decay, because of improper installation. Some dentists avoid using posterior composite fillings because they are more expensive, take more time to place and are often not covered by insurance.

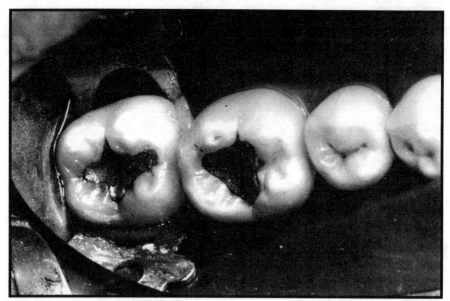

Figure 10.1 Amalgam Restorations

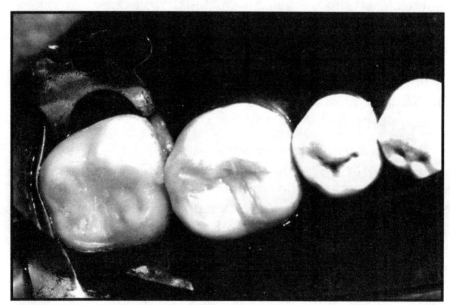

Figure 10.2 Composite Restorations

COMPOSITES: INDIRECT VERSUS DIRECT:

Composites can be placed in an indirect or direct manner. The most common method of placing a composite is directly in the mouth. The tooth is prepared to receive the composite. An etching agent is used to create microscopic tentacles in the enamel and dentin which will grab onto the thin layer of liquid bonding agent which is flowed into the preparation. To this bonding agent, a paste of composite is added and built up in layers to restore the missing tooth structure. As each layer is added, a photosensitive chemical reaction is initiated with a high-intensity light to harden or "cure" the material.

During this whole process, moisture control is critical, thereby necessitating the use of a rubber dam whenever possible. The dam isolates the teeth, affords better visibility, and helps keep saliva away. In my more than 20 years of experience in placing composites, I find that when correctly placed, they are long-lasting and wear-resistant in the vast majority of mouths. The key is to take the necessary time to properly prepare and restore the tooth, and to be extremely exacting.

In the indirect method, the tooth is prepared and an impression of the prepared tooth is taken. An impression of the opposing teeth is also taken, so the functional relationship between the two is recorded. A temporary filling is placed and the impression is sent to a laboratory. There, plaster will be poured into the impression, resulting in an accurate model of the prepared tooth. On this model, the composite restoration is fabricated. It is hardened with light, heat and pressure, yielding a highly-cured, wear-resistant restoration. The advantage of the indirect versus the direct, is that because of the curing method, there will be fewer free chemicals left after the setting reaction. This may be of importance in a highly chemically sensitive individual.

Also because of the method of cure, the wear resistance is higher in the indirect technique, than it is in the direct technique - which may be of value when replacing large areas of chewing surface on a back tooth.

CHAPTER 11

ROOT CANALS

I was taught that the criterion of good dentistry and a good dentist was how many teeth can be saved. Extract a tooth? NEVER! Shame a patient, threaten them with all the problems associated with the loss of a tooth - but do not let a tooth be removed. Just give me a root to work with, and after root canal, gum surgery, a post and a crown and a few thousand dollars, I could look back with amazement at all that modern dentistry could do.

Do not be fooled. I now rank root canals right behind mercury amalgam fillings as a cause of ill health, and with an estimated 60 million root canals performed in 1998, you can appreciate the scope of the problem.

The more experience I gain as a Whole Body Dentist, the more I dread having patients with root canals come to me for evaluation. Although it is understandable, they do not like to hear that all the money, pain and time spent on the root canal may have been a waste - and may even be causing some of their health problems.

Earlier in my career, I was an avid "root canaler", but I soon learned first hand the danger associated with root canals. The wife of a colleague of mine was having chronic kidney problems. My colleague related his wife's experience with Dr. Voll. She had no mercury fillings, but one root canal. Dr. Voll used his electro-acupuncture equipment (known as EAV - *see chapter 21).* to test her energetic pathways and told her she must have the root canal tooth removed. She resisted and tried many other treatments over a period of time. She finally relented, removed the root canal, and her kidney problems completely vanished. When I heard that, I decided it was time to learn more about root canals. And the more I learned the more I was shocked into re-evaluation of this highly intrusive procedure.

ROOT CANAL PROCEDURE:

To appreciate why root canals can be so dangerous, you need to understand the process. A root canal is the removal of the pulpal tissue from the "hollow tube" within the root(s) of the tooth. This pulp is comprised of nerve, blood, and lymphatic tissue. Modern dentists have been taught to "sterilize" the canal of the tooth in this process to ensure that bacteria are not left behind. The canal is then packed with a gummy material called gutta-percha which supposedly seals off the canal. The assumption is held that if you completely sterilize the canal, before sealing it, then a quarantined area exists free from further decay or infection. It makes sense, sounds logical, and dentists have been doing it without a second thought for years. Unfortunately, the process completely ignores the actual physical properties of teeth. (*See the diagram of the tooth Figure 4.1, page 41*)

A tooth's dentin, the material between the enamel or cementum and the canal, is comprised of literally millions of tiny tubules. These tubules exist to transport nutrients from the center of the tooth, through the dentin or cementum to the enamel. And although we think of tooth enamel as a hard and impenetrable material, in reality it is made up of thousands of microscopic tubules. It is living tissue that does indeed allow the passage of fluids and nutrients from the saliva into the tooth and from the dentin out of the tooth.

The dentin is composed of so many of the tiny tubules that if the tubules in your small lower front tooth were laid out end

DENTAL DETECTIVE STORY
CHRONIC SINUS INFECTION FROM ROOT CANALS

Marge was referred to me by a naturopath. A root canal had been done on her upper right first molar 18 months previously. Since that time she had chronic sinus infections and felt constant pressure in the right cheek area. She had been referred by her treating dentist to the head of the Endodontic Department at a well-known dental school.

Both her dentist and the root canal specialist told her that the root canal looked fine and could not possibly be the cause of her problems. They referred her to an ear, nose and throat doctor. Upon his recommendation, a CAT scan was taken which showed the right sinus to be completely infected. Surgery was performed to clean out the sinus.

Marge felt well for about two weeks; then her sinus became infected again. She came to me in desperation, not wanting to undergo another surgery. After consulting with me, Marge decided we should remove the root-canaled tooth.

I called her the next day to see how she was feeling. She was happy to report that she had not experienced any swelling or pain from the removal; but she wanted to ask me something. Was it actually possible for the sinus pressure to go away as quickly as five minutes after the extraction? She felt the pressure disappear right after the procedure - but she was having a hard time believing that it could actually happen that fast! I assured her that not only was it possible for this to happen, but obviously it *did* happen - and that she should relax and trust the successful results. To this day, Marge continues to be without chronic sinus pain or pressure.

to end, it is estimated that they would stretch three miles. It is absurd to believe that these millions of tiny tubules could possibly be "sterilized" during the process of inserting gutta-percha. And even if the tubules could be sterilized, fluid will still move through the enamel, the cementum and the dentin into the canal of the tooth.

Now remember, the canal has been partially sealed with the gutta-percha, so the area no longer benefits from the constant cleansing and oxygenating effect of the blood supply flowing through the tooth. When the bacteria left behind in the dentinal tubules get cut off from the normal oxygen and blood supply in this manner, they begin to metabolize differently. They change from an aerobic to an anaerobic process and begin to give off toxins.

DR. PRICE'S FINDINGS:

If your immune system is strong, your body may be able to quarantine the toxins by "walling off" the area. This may appear on an X-ray as a more radiolucent area indicating an abscess. Dr. Weston Price[*] did 25 years of research on the root canal issue at the beginning of the 20th century. He was taught - and it is still taught today - that a radiolucent area is a bad sign. In fact, as Dr. Price showed, this is the response to the toxins coming from a root-canaled tooth of someone with a good immune system.

Sometimes the reaction is so good that a "drain" will open into the mouth through the gum. Interestingly, when this occurs, there will be no ill effect on the patient. One physician-patient who is in excellent health, as an experiment, has left a draining tooth in place for a number of years.

---

[*] *Dr. Price was a dentist, and one of the foremost researchers of his time. Director of the Research Institute of the National Dental Association, Dr. Price published the 700 page "Dental Infections, Oral and Systemic", and the 400 Page "Dental Infections and the Degenerative Diseases". Both dealt with the effects of root canal teeth on systemic health. Dr. Price is truly one of the "giants" of medicine and dentistry.*

More concern should be given to those teeth seemingly not eliciting any response. If your immune system cannot react quickly or effectively enough to quarantine these bacteria, then their toxins enter your body as negative agents - which attack your genetically weak systems, or your areas of stress. What is interesting about these bacteria, most often a form of a streptococcus, is that they are always present in the mouth. However, when their environment changes after a root canal, in order to survive they mutate and become very toxic. On an X-ray this will appear as a denser area of bone around the root, called a "condensing osteitis."

This problem was first recognized and documented by Dr. Weston Price. His research showed that not only were the medical doctrines and assumptions about root canals incorrect, but that infections following root canals could actually cause the onset of degenerative disease. These root canaled teeth acted as a focus, meaning that they "seed" an infection at a distant site.

In fact, in one study Dr. Price removed root canaled teeth from patients who had developed heart disease following a root canal procedure. Following the extraction, the patients' heart disease "miraculously" improved.

Even more incriminating evidence followed when the extracted root canaled teeth were subsequently implanted in healthy rabbits and they immediately developed heart disease and died. In additional studies, Dr. Price demonstrated how potent and insidious this effect could be by grinding up the teeth, sterilizing the powder, and putting it through a filter to remove all bacteria. Only, and after all that, was a minuscule amount injected into the rabbits - yet still they died of heart disease.

How could that be? Because the bacteria generated in root canaled teeth produce toxins that are virtually indestructible. Dr. Price's extensive research on root canals spanned a period of approximately twenty-five years in the early 1900's, prior to the discovery of antibiotics. This lent a purity to his research since symptoms were clearly displayed and not altered by antibiotics or other drugs.

Because of the raging debate among medical and dental professionals during the years of Dr. Price's research as to the validity of focal infections, Price's work was largely ignored. Today the idea of focal infection is universally accepted. Also, Dr. Percey Howe did a study where he injected rabbits with an oral streptococcus and found no adverse reaction. This study was used by the foes of the focal infection theory to discredit Dr. Price. But remember, these oral bacteria usually are not harmful until they mutate in an anaerobic environment like that in a root canal tooth. Unfortunately, what also occurred was wholesale extraction of teeth by some dentists, trying to cure all and everything. Naturally, this did not happen, but it did tend to discredit the idea of focal infection. This is a lesson we must learn from; we must not think that extraction of teeth is the panacea for all illness.

Dr. George Meinig is one of the founders of the American Association of Endodontics. In a recent book, **Root Canal Cover-Up,**[15] he documents Price's original research, highlighting the striking number of problems and hazards associated with the root-canal procedure. Dr. Meinig also presents research which shows that when gutta-percha, the most widely utilized filling material used in root canals, cools and hardens it shrinks significantly enough for bacteria to enter the tooth and flourish.

To further complicate and compound these problems, it is common after a root canal to do restorative work on the tooth. This usually includes a stainless steel post and core that go into the root of the tooth and comes up into the tooth's crown (the visible part of the tooth). Some dentists will build up the tooth with amalgam and then place a metal or porcelain-to-metal crown over this buildup. This puts dissimilar metals together creating a whole other set of problems as previously discussed in Chapter six. **Root Canal Cover-Up** extensively discusses this topic.

Should all root-canal teeth be removed? Some holistic dentists believe that they should. However, I feel that the human body is too complex to look at this question in black and white.

With the toxicity of the surrounding bone, it is crucial upon extraction of a root-canaled tooth to thoroughly remove the bone surrounding the socket, or there is an increased chance of a subsequent cavitation forming. I have found that using EAV at the time of surgery is the best way to know when this cleansing has been accomplished. Also, let us not forget the work of Dr. Voll, who discovered that root canals also create disturbing *energetic* roadblocks in the body which short- circuit essential pathways leading to the breakdown of proper organ function.

REMOVE ALL ROOT CANALS?

Should all root-canal teeth be removed? Some holistic dentists believe that they all should be removed. However, I feel that the human body is too complex to look at this question in black and white. If a person has a strong immune system, they may be able to tolerate a root-canal. I think a lot also has to do with the meridian the tooth is on. For example, if the person has a weak liver, a root canal performed on the canine tooth which is on the liver meridian, will be more problematic. Conversely, balancing the chemistry and strengthening the liver may allow a person to handle a previously toxic root canal. I have seen patients who have three root canaled teeth, but only one is not being tolerated. Dr. Price showed that inoculating rabbits from root-canaled teeth obtained from asymptomatic individuals usually did not produce any symptoms. Human beings have many compensatory mechanisms, and to say that all root canal teeth must be removed in all people is too extreme. I have found EAV is the best way to evaluate what the root canals are doing and for periodically monitoring them, especially if a person's health has changed.

What is important is that the patient be educated with reference to root canals, so that they can make an informed decision. Also they need to know that a root canal tooth which is currently being tolerated may at some future time become intolerable, due to age, accident or illness.

Dr. Price did show that in many individuals with any kind of history of degenerative disease in their family, the root canal procedure actually caused the onset of that disease in an otherwise healthy patient. Factoring in your family health history is definitely one of the things that must enter into the decision of whether or not to have a root canal. Also, you must consider your health at the time of making a decision. If you are chronically ill at the time of needing a root canal, extraction may be the better choice.

Most often, my treatment will initially evaluate the root canal's systemic effect; but I urge the patient not to make any decisions until their chemistry is balanced and their overall toxicity is addressed.

RECENT RESEARCH INTO ROOT CANALS:

At the University of Kentucky, Drs. Boyd Haley and Curt Pendergrass have conducted research into the toxicity of root-canaled teeth. These researchers have devised an ingenious method of testing: they take extracted root canal teeth and dip them into a beaker of sterile water. This is done three times, each time in a new beaker of sterile water. A sample of water from the third dipping is then tested against several critical human enzyme systems. Depending upon the amount of inhibition of the enzymes, they rate whether a tooth is severely, extremely, moderately, mildly or slightly toxic. Some teeth which have been tested have been among the most toxic materials the researchers have ever seen. They call this ALT testing. The ALT stands for Affinity Labeling Technology. This type of testing can also be done with tissue samples from cavitations (*see Chapter 13*).

The enzymes they have chosen are all involved in the production of ATP. Every cellular process depends upon ATP (Adenosin triphosphate). Therefore anything which interferes with ATP production is detrimental. What becomes critical is where the toxin accumulates. For example, if the toxins accumulate in the heart tissue, enzyme inhibition will occur which may become severe enough to impair proper heart function. Where the toxins accumulate, and hence their effect, is not addressed by this testing.

Because their testing showed different levels of toxicity of extracted root canal teeth, Drs. Haley and Pendergrass then devised a testing procedure to evaluate root-canal teeth still in the mouth - thus helping a patient make the decision to extract or not to extract. A sterile paper point is placed in the space between the tooth and the gum (the "sulcus") next to the root canal, to absorb some of the fluid present. A control sample is taken from around a healthy tooth, with healthy gum tissue, at a site distant from the root canal. These fluid samples are then tested to determine the degree of toxicity present. Because there are toxins normally present in the mouth, it is very important to use the patient's

DENTAL DETECTIVE STORY
A KIDNEY CONNECTION?

A patient was referred in because his wife had read about the effect of mercury on the kidneys. Her husband was now on dialysis awaiting a kidney transplant. The patient's concern was that, because the doctors had no idea why his kidneys had shut down, what was to stop the transplanted kidney from also malfunctioning? Upon EAV testing it was discovered that mercury was not the main problem. The real interference was a root canal on an upper front tooth, which coincidentally is on the kidney meridian. Testing from the University of Kentucky was then performed, with the results showing severe toxicity of the root canaled tooth compared to the control. Armed with this information and knowing that the surgeons had said to get rid of any mouth infection, he decided to extract the tooth. I also referred him to a physician to test his mercury levels.

own control sample for comparison. Experience with this procedure has shown that there is a strong correlation of the tested levels of toxicity before extraction, and after extraction of the tooth.

Just very recently, an inexpensive ALT test has been devised for use in the dental office. The five minute test will screen root canal teeth for toxicity. Those screening as toxic can be further tested with the ususal ALT test.

BIOCALEX:

Traditionally, root-canaled teeth have been sealed with gutta-percha. This gummy substance contracts with time, thus creating spaces between the dentin and the gutta-percha, thereby allowing bacteria present in the blood stream to enter the tooth. A product to seal root canals that has been used in Europe for a number of years is called BioCalex. This is a calcium oxide material which upon setting in the tooth expands and forms calcium hydroxide and calcium carbonate. The resulting material is very alkaline, thereby tending to create an environment which hinders bacterial growth. Also, because of the expansion upon setting, a tight seal between the material and the tooth is obtained.

Limited testing up to this point at the University of Kentucky has shown a dramatic decrease in toxicity of BioCalex treated teeth, versus those treated with gutta-percha. Long-term research continues.

In testing with EAV, thus far I have noticed a higher level of tolerance in BioCalex treated teeth. Not having been able to test many teeth treated with BioCalex, especially after they have been in place for a few years, the jury is still out. However, if in fact they are rendering the tooth less toxic than those done with gutta-percha, it will be easier for the body to compensate. In fact, I tell patients that being in good health, if I had a tooth die, I would do a Bio-Calex root canal and then monitor it with EAV.

CHAPTER 12

IMPLANTS - AN ALTERNATIVE TO ROOT CANALS

I mplants are titanium rods which are placed into the jawbone in an area where a tooth is missing. The bone then solidifies around the rod. A crown is then placed upon the part of the rod that protrudes into the mouth. Implants are big business today, with many dentists very often recommending implants rather than a bridge after a tooth is extracted. For people not having a back tooth on which to anchor a bridge, an implant can be a marvelous option. But, are they safe?

I personally have not had the opportunity to test a large number of implants with EAV. The ones I have tested have shown mixed results, with some testing poorly and others testing very well. Like root canals, some holistic dentists believe that all implants are detrimental. However, as with root canals, I believe the individual's state of health, genetics and reserve capacity will determine whether they are safe or not for that particular individual. Again, the health of the specific meridian on which the implant is being placed is critical. It would also be a good idea to have compatibility testing to check for specific implant materials by brand name.

In discussing implant options with patients, one area of concern is the electrical component. I believe that there is a better chance of tolerating a titanium implant if it is placed in a mouth that has no other metals. Ideally, there should be no amalgams or other metals in the mouth. Also, the crowns being placed upon the implant should be made of a composite or porcelain, in order to lessen the electrical impact of the implant upon the body. Compatibility testing also checks for suitable implants by brand name for the particular individual.

CHAPTER 13

CAVITATIONS

Cavitations are a relatively new term in the dental dialogue. Most patients are not aware of cavitations, and even most dentists probably do not know much about them as yet.

WHAT ARE CAVITATIONS?

A cavitation is a hole in the bone, usually where a tooth has been removed and the bone has not filled in properly. When a tooth is being extracted, in what has been normal dental procedure, the surrounding periodontal membrane is usually left behind. Theoretically, when a tooth has been pulled, the body will eventually fill in the space in the bone where the tooth once was. But when the membrane is left behind, an incomplete healing can take place which leaves a hole or a spongy place inside the jaw bone. Experts speculate that perhaps this is because the bone cells on either side sense the presence of the periodontal membrane and "think" that the tooth is still there.

WHERE CAN CAVITATIONS FORM?

A cavitation can form in any bone in the body, not just in the jaw bones. There are also other reasons that cavitations form, some of which are localized traumas, poor circulation to the area, clotting disorders, and the use of steroids.

On X-ray of an extracted tooth site, this membrane can form an image that appears to be a shadow of a tooth. Almost always, this is indicative of a cavitation. Most dentists are aware of this phantom tooth image, but they do not recognize it as a site of potential problems.

WHAT'S HIDING INSIDE?

Inside a cavitation, bacteria flourish and deviant cells multiply. Cavitations act as a breeding ground for bacteria and their toxins. Research has shown these bacterial waste products to be extremely potent. Cavitations can also cause blockages on the body's energy meridians and can exert far-reaching impact on the overall system. Investigation has revealed that some cavitations are reservoirs of huge amounts of mercury. Cavitations may be a source of low level or high level stress on the entire body.

DIAGNOSIS

Diagnosing cavitations is an elusive process because cavitations do not always readily appear on X-rays. Sometimes they show up only as very subtle differentiations in the texture pattern of the bone. If your dentist is not specifically looking for the cavitations, then your X-ray will be read as looking "just fine".

Cavitations may be a source of low-level or high level stress on the entire body. Cavitations can also cause blockages on the body's energy meridians and can exert far-reaching impact on the overall system.

There are other ways to discover cavitation sites. For example, they will sometimes cause pain when the area is lightly stroked or when pressure is applied. The EAV instrument is extremely effective in helping find potential cavitation sites, however it is not recognized as a diagnostic device so the patient must assimilate all the evidence and decide how they want to proceed with treatment. There is a new instrument, similar to a sonogram, which will be coming out soon that will detect these cavitations.

MOST COMMON SITES

The most common place for cavitations is the third molar area - the area where the wisdom teeth are removed, followed by areas of root canal extraction. Because so many of the body's major organs are on the wisdom tooth meridian, cavitations in this area are particularly worrisome. Dr. Voll felt that cavitations in the wisdom tooth area are the major underlying cause of heart problems in later life *(see figure 21.3)*.

Several years ago, I myself developed an arrhythmia which did not correct with vitamin or mineral supplementation, herbs or homeopathy. On EAV evaluation, one cavitation was found in the lower left wisdom tooth area.

DENTAL DETECTIVE STORY
POST EXTRACTION PROBLEMS

Andrea was very nervous when I examined her. She explained that ever since her wisdom tooth was removed, if the tissue in that area was touched, she would experience an extreme shock-like pain in her lip. She also told me she had residual numbness of the lip and gum since the extraction. After seeing her several times, she gained enough confidence to allow me to test the area around the extraction site that was so sensitive to touch. I found a cavitation present and treated it by injecting homeopathic remedies directly into the area. Her numbness disappeared, she is no longer hypersensitive to touch, and she has had no more occurrences of the shock-like pain in her lip.

Surgical debridement of the cavitation resolved the problem in a few days. The wisdom tooth had been extracted twenty-five years earlier! Up until the point of symptoms, evidently my body was able to compensate for the blockage of my energy flow through this meridian.

TREATMENT:

I often recommend two primary methods of treatment for my patients. First is a procedure where special homeopathic medications called Sanum remedies are injected into the cavitation site, and then a modified form of low level laser light therapy is applied to the area. If this method is not successful, the alternative is to surgically open the area and clean the remaining ligament and resultant debris from the bone. Every biopsy of bone material I have collected from cavitation surgeries has shown osteonecrosis, or dead bone material.

NICO:

Specialists have recognized cavitations as a possible cause of chronic facial pain and termed them "NICO" (Neuralgia Inducing Cavitational Osteonecrosis). Often this is the overlooked factor in trigeminal neuralgia, as well as other kinds of facial pain.

SICO:

While it is good that the impact of cavitations on facial pain is finally being considered, the far-reaching bodily impact of cavitations is still vastly underappreciated. Cavitations on major meridians can cause serious health problems. I prefer to call cavitations "SICO", or Sickness Inducing Cavitational Osteonecrosis, which better indicates the power a cavitation can have over the general health of the patient. Analysis of cavitational samples by researchers at the University of Kentucky have thus far found every one of them to contain biologically toxic material.

SURGERY & EAV:

Just before surgery I check which acupuncture meridians are adversely affected by the cavitation. After I have thoroughly debrided the cavitational area, I once again check the acupuncture meridians using EAV. It is fascinating to see how the readings for these meridians will return to normal after the cavitation is properly treated. In fact, if the reading is not normalized, it means more debridement is necessary.

PRECAUTIONS:

While cavitations can be caused by removal of teeth, this does not necessarily mean that you should not have teeth removed. It does mean that if an extraction is necessary, the dentist should clean out the periodontal ligament and any infection that is present,

DENTAL DETECTIVE STORY

COMPLEXION

Rose had problems with acne since she was a teenager. She was now in her late thirties. Rose was referred by a physician, who suspected the presence of cavitations. Four cavitational areas were detected where teeth had been removed for orthodontic treatment when Rose was about twelve. A side benefit of cleaning out these abnormal areas of bone was an acne-free complexion.

as part of the normal procedure. By doing this, the wound will have the greatest chance of healing normally, giving the patient no further difficulty. The healing process will also go more smoothly if the appropriate organ systems are supported homeopathically and/or nutritionally. Before the surgery I also find it beneficial to have the patient take five calcium lactate tablets twice a day for five days. I have them continue this regimen for five days after the procedure.

CHAPTER 14

PERIODONTAL DISEASE

Periodontal disease has practically become a national pastime. Some estimates place more than 85% of the U.S. population over the age of 30 with this disease. Periodontal disease comprises a broad range of problems from gingivitis, a simple inflammation of the gums, to full periodontitis, which involves loss of bone around the teeth.

CAUSES:

There is ample evidence to suggest that bacteria cause periodontal disease - in fact, fluid cultured from the pockets surrounding the affected teeth can be analyzed for a specific strain of bacteria to select the most effective course of antibiotics for treatment. Recently small chips have been developed which can be inserted into a periodontal pocket. These chips slowly release small amounts of antibiotic as the chip resorbs. Also, controlling the level of bacteria by brushing and flossing may be of benefit. But I have found that there is more to periodontal disease than just the bugs.

While the presence of bacteria does play a role, the essential element in whether a person will develop gum disease may actually have much more to do with their general health. We all have bacteria, not only in our mouths, but throughout our bodies. One reason some people develop problems, while others do not, is because the host's resistance is low, providing a prime environment for bacteria to multiply. There are people who do not floss or brush regularly and they have no problems. On the other hand, I have seen patients who are religious about their oral hygiene, practically to the point of neurosis, yet over time gum disease will continue to progress and deteriorate the bone. I know of many individuals who have undergone periodontal surgery, spent thousands of dollars, had their teeth cleaned every three months and still have not arrested the disease.

If I find a generalized periodontal problem, I think more in terms of a systemic problem like mercury toxicity, nutrition and overall body chemistry. If the problem is just in certain localized areas, it is more likely linked to a number of factors related to the tooth including interference on its energetic meridian relating to a specific organ, a defective restoration or crown margin, a very high electrical current, or a bite problem.

YOUR BITE

Proper bite and alignment of the teeth also impacts heavily on the health of the gums. Excessive or improper pressure on the teeth, caused by bite problems, can literally create an environment around the tooth that predisposes it to a bacterial invasion and problems.

Proper bite and alignment of the teeth also impacts heavily on the health of the gums. Excessive or improper pressure on the teeth, caused by bite problems, can literally create an environment around the tooth that predisposes it to a bacterial invasion and problems. A misaligned bite can cause a tooth to become so loose, that the patient fears it may actually fall out. Constant unbalanced pressure on a tooth has a similar effect to someone leaning on and twisting a stake in the ground. With the pressure and movement, the earth supporting the stake begins to move away, or "trough". This same phenomenon occurs to the bone supporting the tooth, and the troughing of the bone provides a direct pathway for bacteria to enter.

What is remarkable is that this localized process is often reversible. By correcting the bite problem and cleaning the area around the tooth on several successive visits, the bone may actually "fill in" around the tooth, holding it tight again. Not only is it important to recognize bite problems as a source of gum dysfunction, it is equally essential that proper attention be given to the bite after any periodontal surgery. A bite adjustment is a meticulous reshaping of the tooth surfaces in order to properly direct the forces on the teeth creating harmonious functioning. Many dentists do not have the specialized training to perform this process effectively. I learned to do proper bite adjustments at the world-renowned Pankey Institute. If you are going to have such work done, you should seek out a dentist who has taken post-graduate courses in this technique.

AMALGAM FILLINGS

The dental specialists who treat gum disease, known as periodontists, do not receive training about many of the holistic factors that affect proper gum health. As usual, the impact of mercury has been overlooked. A major sign of mercury toxicity, bleeding gums and loose teeth, is often mistakenly treated as gum disease. You would be amazed at how many patients' gums stop bleeding after having their mercury amalgam fillings removed.

Studies of tissue adjacent to amalgam fillings show that the mercury and other toxic metals present in the amalgam "leak" into the area causing an inflammatory reaction.

HOST RESISTANCE

A greatly neglected, yet essential element of gum health is the blood which provides the primary nourishment for the gums and bone *(see chapter 25)*. Periodontal disease is a degenerative disease just like diabetes or arthritis. Studies show a correlation between osteoporosis and jaw bone loss. As such, balancing a person's body chemistry plays a large factor in combating this disease. When bacteria confront a strong immune system, they cannot do their "dirty work". Having blood and hair testing is usually a prudent idea when confronted with a case of generalized periodontal disease.

This is the great debate: does bacteria cause disease, or in fact, is it alteration of the host resistance (or "terrain") that allows bacteria to multiply? Depending upon your belief, the thrust of treatment will vary. If bacteria are the cause, then just kill the bacteria with antibiotics or mouthwashes. However, if you believe - as I do - that the terrain is the critical factor, then treatment is directed towards alteration of the host's resistance. To this end, the use of hair and blood analysis is essential in guiding proper nutrition and supplementation on an individual basis.

During the course of ten years, my father suffered from periodontal disease and underwent numerous surgical procedures. He was diligent in his home care, brushing and flossing regularly. Despite doing everything "by the book" to arrest the disease, he continued to develop pockets and lose bone. As I began to learn more about the functioning of the human system and how the blood and immune system can impact gum disease, I would share the information with him. He changed his eating habits and supplemented his diet and enjoyed a considerable improvement in his blood "quality". His periodontal disease ceased troubling him and he has not had a problem or a symptom now

---

DENTAL DETECTIVE STORY
TOXIC PERIODONTAL POCKETS

Ralph, 56 years old, was referred by a physician for a thorough dental exam. He owned a factory and was upset that his health problems were interfering with his ability to work. He had a terrible left shoulder pain, general malaise, and could not think clearly. He had not felt well for several years. At this point, one of his children was running the business on a daily basis. Ralph had two upper left molars with extremely deep pockets - approximately 12 millimeters. I told Ralph the teeth were hopeless and needed to be extracted.

EAV testing showed these teeth to be adversely affecting several acupuncture meridians. I guess the toxins from these teeth were literally infecting his entire system, because one week after removal Ralph was a new man. His energy had sky rocketed, his mind was sharp, and he felt ten years younger.

---

in more than twenty years. An additional side benefit was that his formerly high cholesterol became normalized and he was able to stop using cholesterol lowering drugs. He was once again able to enjoy eating eggs - and with a healthy mouth!

GUM SURGERY:

Sometimes surgery to reduce the pocket depth is necessary. Periodontists today have new and exciting surgical techniques available. Previously, periodontal treatment involved taking away infected gum or bone. Today, they can often restore and build up the bone level. However, I usually suggest that my patients try a non-surgical approach first. This involves balancing their chemistry and meticulous home care, as well as cleaning out the existing pockets. In general natural Vitamin C and Co-Enzyme Q-10 are particularly helpful. I also recommend irrigating the pockets with a very high quality herbal product called Tooth and Gum Tonic. This kills the bacteria, helps soothe inflammation, and is a connective tissue conditioner and rebuilder.

Just like a root canal or an impacted tooth, a periodontal pocket could actually be causing disturbances in other areas of the body.

Many patients ask me how to properly brush their teeth to ward off gum disease. Up and down, side to side, or in circles are some of the popular variations, but it really does not matter all that much. As long as you use a soft brush and brush <u>at the gum line,</u> whatever style you are comfortable with should be adequate to the task. If you like to use an electric brush, I have seen great results with the Rotadent, which can only be purchased through your dentist.

As with any other problem with the teeth, it is essential to recognize and appreciate the energetic relationship to the rest of the body. Periodontal disease, bite problems, and resulting surgery can be impacted by and have tremendous impact on other areas of the body. Just like a root canal or an impacted tooth, a periodontal pocket could actually be causing disturbances in other areas of the body *(see chapter 21).*

I find interesting the recent newspaper headlines which cite studies correlating a higher incidence of heart disease in those with periodontal disease. They advocate treating the periodontal disease to prevent heart problems, because bacteria associated with gum inflammation are also associated with heart disease. However, no one discusses the possibility that the same underlying body chemistry imbalance is really the common denominator in both heart and gum disease.

CHAPTER 15

CROWNS

A crown, or cap, is a sheath of metal fitted over a carved-down tooth, usually done in cases where the tooth has decayed to the degree that it would take a very large filling to repair the tooth. Very often crowns are necessary for mercury-filled teeth because the mercury weakens the tooth and fractures occur. Crowns are made in a dental laboratory, necessitating impressions and the use of temporary crowns while the permanent crowns are being fabricated.

GOLD CROWNS:

MERCURY RELEASE

Gold is normally a very good material for crowns, but there is one exception: you should never put a gold crown in a mouth with amalgam fillings. The gold will speed up the release of mercury from the amalgams, so that your body burden of mercury will increase faster than it would with just amalgams alone. A more aesthetic choice is porcelain bonded to gold, but there is still the problem of having gold in the same mouth with amalgams.

ELECTRICAL PROBLEMS

If you need a crown and do not want to have your amalgams removed, you should only have a porcelain or composite crown placed. Of course, the traditional gold crown carries with it the

DENTAL DETECTIVE STORY

PROBLEM FROM A CROWN

Peter, a 32-year-old man, came in for a dental examination. Upon initial cancer screening I found that the gums were very inflamed around an upper left molar crown, especially on the tongue side of the mouth. I referred the patient to a periodontist for consultation because something just did not look right.

The periodontist did a biopsy and the tissue was cancerous. He related to me, that in his experience, in every case of cancer around a tooth with a crown, the crown was nickel based. This case was no different (nickel is carcinogenic).

possible significant health hazard of having any metal in the mouth, along with the resultant electrical currents.

OTHER METALS

Worse than gold in the mouth is having some other kind of metal or porcelain-to-metal crown. As dentists we have license to place an assortment of toxic metals, like nickel or palladium.

PRESERVING TOOTH STRUCTURE:

I try to avoid using crowns since they require a lot of tooth mutilation - which dramatically increases the odds of needing a root canal in the future. I also try to avoid onlays. Onlays are restorations that cover the cusps of the teeth but do not remove tooth structure down to the gum, like a crown. Instead, I try to save as much of the tooth as possible by using bondable materials. Teeth that I would have thought needed crowns or onlays in the past, I now usually can restore in a much more conservative manner. Twenty years ago I had my mouth restored with gold onlays. If I were doing it today, I would have my teeth restored with composite fillings. I believe that several years from now we may develop the means to "regrow" enamel from any remaining enamel, and this is another good reason to try to save as much of the tooth structure as possible.

I spent my first five years in private practice immersing myself in what is called "full mouth rehabilitation." Consequently, many patients came to me to rebuild their mouths, which resulted in many root canals and lots of gold and placement of crowns and bridges. I was taught to make every mouth "ideal." Over the years, seeing the possibly immense negative impact dentistry may have, I now espouse doing the least amount of dentistry possible, compatible with proper function, esthetics and with the overall well-being of the individual kept uppermost in my mind.

CHAPTER 16

BRIDGES AND PARTIALS

A traditional bridge consists of two supporting teeth with a false tooth in the middle. The bridge is permanently inserted into the mouth, in one piece, to replace a missing tooth or teeth.

BRIDGES:

Until recently, in most instances, when replacing a missing tooth with a bridge, we had no choice but to use full crowns on the supporting teeth. This often resulted in the mutilation of one or two perfectly healthy non restored teeth. New composite materials now allow us to make a non metal bridge without doing full crowns, resulting in minimal damage to the buttressing teeth. Studies indicate that these new substances are as strong as metal. These bridges are bonded to the supporting teeth and are not removable.

PARTIALS:

A partial is a removable false-tooth appliance which anchors on either side of the mouth, by "clasping" some of the remaining teeth. These clasps often place a large amount of stress on the

DENTAL DETECTIVE STORY

ELECTRICAL PHENOMENON

A patient of mine was exposed to a chemical material which left him highly allergic and very electrically sensitive. Fluorescent lights bothered him; he would get shooting pains down his arms while driving a car; and he often had joint pains. He had a metal partial and a mouth full of amalgam fillings. We began treatment by removing the fillings and his symptoms were considerably lessened - most of his joint pain entirely disappeared, and he was able to drive again. However, he continued to experience a strange phenomenon.

Every so often, he would be outdoors when suddenly he would be jolted so strongly that he literally would think that he got hit by a bolt of lightening. After several of these incidents, he finally realized that it always happened when a large airplane went overhead. He came back to me with this bizarre story.

We did an Electrodermal (refer to chapter 21) screening on his nervous system meridian, first with him wearing the metal partial and then with it removed. There was a profound difference in the functioning of his nervous system in these two tests. I told him to stop wearing the partial for a while to see if it was the culprit. Sure enough, the strange occurrence ceased. We made him a new, all plastic partial and he is now fine. We may never know what odd phenomenon was taking place, but I will certainly never underestimate the potential dangers of having such a large plate of metal in the mouth.

teeth. Generally there is a metal plate that runs across the hard palate on an upper partial, or along the back of the lower front teeth for a lower partial.

A metal partial is particularly offensive, because it places a large metal surface with a large electrical component in the head. With some upper metal partials, the plate runs across the top of the mouth immobilizing the center suture of the craniosacral system.

DENTAL DETECTIVE STORY
SHOULDER PAIN FROM A BRIDGE

Cavitations and root canals are not the only elements that can produce a focus -, i.e., send a signal that is picked up at a remote site in the body and causes a problem. Sometimes a symptom as innocuous as an ill-fitting bridge can be a problem.

Eleanor came to see me for a routine dental exam. Upon taking her history I discovered that she had a chronic pain in her right shoulder. Otherwise, she was in good health. I also noted that she had a bridge in the lower right side of her mouth where the tissue was very inflamed and bled easily. It was not causing her any pain in her mouth, but because the bridge was very unaesthetic, she asked to have it replaced. Surprisingly, after the bridge was removed and the tissue healed, her chronic shoulder problem went away.

Plastic partials are available and highly advisable, especially if there are other metals already present in the mouth. The new materials available for nonmetal partials have clasps that flex, resulting in less stress on the supporting teeth. The cranial sutures are also allowed normal movement. Thus far, my patients that have opted for these new partials have expressed their satisfaction with them. However, wherever possible, I would recommend a fixed bridge. It is more stable and gives better chewing efficiency.

CHAPTER 17

THE GREAT AMERICAN HEADACHE

Headaches have practically become a national pastime; they are the seventh leading complaint in outpatient medical care in the U.S. During the past year, nearly 90% of men and 95% of women have had at least one headache. An estimated 50 million Americans suffer some form of severe headache; they make more than 18 million outpatient visits to physicians every year for this condition, according to the American Association for the Study of Headache. Twenty six-million Americans suffer from migraine - about 12% of our population as a whole.

What most people, physicians included, do not realize is that *a tremendous number of these headaches are related to the teeth.* In my experience, as much as 85% of all head pain has been directly attributable to problems in the teeth and jaw - and it is readily alleviated with proper dental treatment.

When my new receptionist told me she had been getting headaches nearly every day for several years, I immediately suspected a problem with her teeth. Sure enough her wisdom teeth were impacted. Since she never had any specific problems with them, she did not know that they needed to come out. And once they were removed? You guessed it - 99% of her headaches have completely vanished. She does still report an occasional headache, but we have both come to the conclusion that once her three kids are a bit older, those will probably also miraculously vanish!

DENTAL DETECTIVE STORY
HEAD PAIN FROM TMD

Dorothy was referred to me by her acupuncturist. She had constant pain on the right side of her head which began immediately after having a filling placed in her upper right molar two years previously. To Dorothy, it felt like the pain was coming from that tooth. She had been examined by several dentists and physicians but no cause could be uncovered.

It seemed to me that if Dorothy felt the pain was coming from the filling, it did not matter if we could "uncover" a medical reason for the pain - we should JUST remove the restoration and see what happens. With her permission, I removed the amalgam and replaced it with a medicated filling - a temporary material that releases a soothing medication into the tooth. Unfortunately that did not relieve the pain.

I had also noticed that Dorothy bit her nails and suspected that it could be triggering a TMD problem. To keep her from biting her nails, I made a small plastic appliance that went over her upper front teeth. In very short order, the pain went away. The appliance also helped Dorothy to break the nail biting habit. She is now pain free and no longer needs to wear the appliance.

TENSION HEADACHES:

The result of stress, tension headaches are the most common, afflicting as many as 75% of all headache sufferers. Ninety percent of all adults have had a tension headache, says the American Council for Headaches. Tension headaches are usually a steady ache rather than a throbbing pain; they affect both sides of the head. I believe psychological factors have been greatly overemphasized as a cause of tension headaches.

You might think that the only way to treat a tension headache would be to reduce the amount of tension or learn how to "relax" more, but that is not always possible or even easily accomplished. It is also not the only answer.

MISALIGNED BITE

Many times people under stress will clench or grind their teeth, which is frequently the result of a misaligned bite. As a result, the tension headache is almost always accompanied by spasms of the muscles which help to open and close the jaw. To evaluate whether the headaches are bite related, we make a small mold fitting over the upper front teeth, which the patient wears for several days. Often, the headaches stop entirely or diminish greatly. We then know to go ahead and make minor, but important, adjustments to reshape the teeth so the patient can have long lasting relief. When the bite is corrected, the strain is taken off the muscles which are free to relax and heal, while the patient continues to feel better and better.

TMD - TEMPOROMANDIBULAR DYSFUNCTION:

TMD - formerly known as TMJ syndrome - is simply a dramatic extension of the classic tension headache. It is named for the Temporomandibular Joint which is in front of the ear where the lower jaw rests in the skull bone socket. Often related to clenching and misaligned bite, over time the TMD syndrome can result in extreme spasms and trauma to the muscles not only in the jaw, but down into the neck and shoulders. In many cases, even the back muscles are affected.

Between the top of the lower jaw, called the condyle, and the skull, is a cartilaginous disc. This serves as a cushion as the condyle moves forward and down when the mouth is opening. If this gets displaced slightly, there will occur a click or pop upon opening the mouth; sometimes the jaw may even lock (*see figure 17.1*).

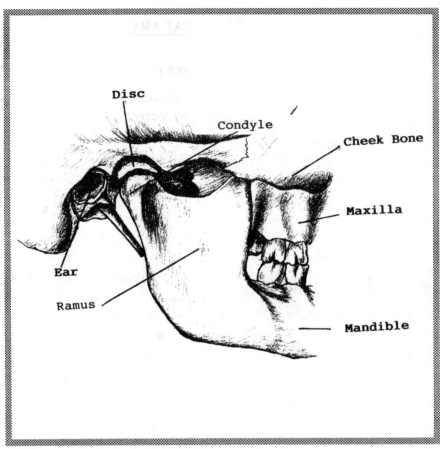

Figure 17.1 Drawing of Skull

SYMPTOMS

Some symptoms of TMD include dizziness, headaches, migraines, facial pain, tooth pain, pain down the arms into the fingers, lack of jaw opening, pain upon jaw movement, ringing in the ears, grinding of the teeth and chronic neck and backache.

ENERGY MERIDIANS

Since the site of the Temporomandibular Joint is at the intersection of three major energy meridians relating to the stomach, endocrine system and small intestine, relief of TMD can spark a tremendous healing process in the whole body, relieving symptoms like stomach problems, chest pains and cold extremities.

BITE ADJUSTMENT

TMD generally requires bite adjustments (reshaping of the tooth surfaces) and sometimes braces to correct the misalignment. And because TMD causes so much trauma to the whole system and especially the skeletal structure and muscles, I will often recommend a homeopathic remedy and bodywork to hasten the healing process during or after the bite adjustment process.

Since the site of the Temporomandibular Joint is at the intersection of the three major energy meridians relating to the stomach, endocrine system and small intestine, relief of TMD can spark a tremendous healing process in the whole body, relieving symptoms like stomach problems, chest pains and cold extremities.

Sometimes prior to the bite adjustment, or while treatment is in progress, an appliance is needed. This goes over either the upper or lower teeth, to reposition the jaw thereby alleviating the muscle spasms.

DIFFICULT CASES

Not all TMD is remedied by correcting the bite, and sometimes the improvement is limited. I became curious as to why only certain cases of TMD would respond and began to notice that the "difficult" cases often occurred in patients who had mercury amalgam fillings with high electrical readings. My hypothesis is that these metals were emitting enough electricity in the oral cavity to interfere with proper muscle functioning and with the local energy meridians. Sure enough, when the fillings were removed, many patients experienced tremendous relief. Remarkably, much of the time, removal of the metals in the mouth was all that was required to alleviate the symptoms of TMD.

Patients that had traditional orthodontics with extraction of teeth were often more of a problem and frequently needed orthodontic retreatment (*see chapter 18*).

DENTAL DETECTIVE STORY
MISALIGNED BITE

Rachel, a woman in her mid-forties, came in with her husband. She had such bad migraines that she was unable to drive. Since they had the financial resources, they had been all over the country looking for help. She had classic migraine symptoms of photosensitivity, vomiting, and severe pain, and would often spend a number of days in bed when a migraine struck.

Upon examination, I found her bite to be misaligned and all her chewing muscles in extremely acute spasm. An appliance was made to correct her bite. This relieved the muscle spasms and her migraines disappeared.

This was then followed by reshaping her own teeth so that she could then go without the appliance. Nutritional support was also provided. In the approximately 15 years since treatment she has been fine, needing just a few minor readjustments.

DENTAL PARAMETERS

About 23 years ago I was called before the dental board because I was treating patients with headaches related to their bite. The board objected to a dentist treating headaches but I was able to convince them I was treating the underlying cause of the headache which was, indeed, within the parameters of dentistry.

Now, there are a lot of standard accepted treatments for TMD which include extensive reconstructive work or years of orthodontics. You may be able to obtain the same results in terms of relieving symptoms in a far less intrusive manner. It is always advisable, though, to look at the symptoms in context of all the different factors before making treatment decisions.

TRIGEMINAL NEURALGIA (TN):

TN, a frequently misunderstood problem, is easy to misdiagnose since the pain comes on suddenly and lasts only a few seconds. TN is marked by a sharp pain that usually starts at one side of the mouth and "shoots-out" to the lips, gums, cheek, ear, eye, or nostril on the affected side. The pain is truly terrible and has resulted in suicide in some cases; it recurs frequently and can be triggered by touch, movement, eating, and even by very subtle changes in temperature like a draft of air.

Often people under stress will clench or grind their teeth, which is frequently the result of a misaligned bite. As a result, the tension headache is almost always accompanied by spasms of the muscles which help to open and close the jaw.

A syndrome similar to TN results in atypical facial pain. This is a constant, often burning pain, which affects one side of the face and can include discomfort in the head and neck as well. This facial pain is not "triggered" suddenly like TN, and the pain may spread beyond the affected side of the face.

Minor cases of TN and atypical facial pain cause minimal, yet nearly constant discomfort, and many patients simply live with the symptoms often with drugs keeping the pain under control. More pronounced cases are usually treated by a neurologist. Expensive diagnostic tests often fail to determine an underlying cause or cure.

Very often, I find TN and atypical facial pain are the result of dental procedures. Frequently the pain is from a cavitation. The drilling of a very tiny hole into the cavitation, followed by

DENTAL DETECTIVE STORY

FACIAL PAIN

Helen was referred to me by a naturopathic physician.

Her head was covered by a scarf; she could not easily wash or brush her hair because of the excruciating pain this would trigger. Any draft of air on her face would also cause her terrible pain. Her teeth had not been cleaned in years because cleaning procedures in her mouth would also set off the pain. Needless to say, she was at wit's end.

The pain went from her lower jaw, up to the side and back of her head. She was on medication, which gave some relief but not much - just enough to keep her from committing suicide.

When I examined her, I found that she had multiple bridges, amalgams, and cavitations. The amalgams were removed and the cavitations treated, which resulted in substantial relief. Not thinking that removal of the crowns and bridges would help, I cautioned against that procedure because I thought it might be a waste of money.

Helen, however, insisted that we remove all the metals, and this gave her even more relief. Although she is not 100% better, she is about 95% improved - and no longer has that excruciating pain. She can comfortably wash her hair and have her teeth cleaned.

the injection of a few drops of anesthetic, will immediately demonstrate if the pain is really emanating from this area. Sometimes the case can be complicated, with the pain having cavitational, electrical, and bite components.

A FEW WORDS OF CAUTION:

If you experience sudden or chronic head pain, have a physician rule out tumors, high blood pressure, etc. If no underlying medical problem can be found, before starting with suppressive drug therapy, see a dentist trained in TMD treatment.

CHAPTER 18

ORTHODONTICS

I can spot someone who has had traditional orthodontics a mile away. There is a typical orthodontic look - almost as though something is awry in the structural composition of the face and jaw. Often people look as though their mouth is "bashed in" instead of in balance with the rest of their face and head. That is because some orthodontists move teeth around without considering the relationship of the jaw to the surrounding cranial system. If you stop to think about it, your common sense will tell you that you cannot change the shape of your mouth without affecting the rest of your head.

Unfortunately not all orthodontists are trained to think this way. A lot of orthodontic treatment is done without regard to the rest of the head and face, with terrible results. For example, it is common practice to move "buck" teeth back to correct the bite. But the problem with buck teeth is usually not that they stick out too far - it is that the bottom jaw does not extend out far enough. Proper whole body dental treatment calls for the jaw to be brought forward into balance with the whole structure of the head.

BICUSPID EXTRACTION:

Usually extraction of the bicuspids is done to give room to allow the upper front teeth to be drawn back. The bicuspids are the teeth just behind the eye teeth. When I began seeing a lot of TMD patients, I noticed that many of them had their bicuspids removed at an early age. There are numerous disadvantages and problems associated with this: the first and foremost is a functional change in the temporomandibular joint apparatus. I firmly believe that orthodontics and bicuspid removal greatly contribute to the onset of TMD. Furthermore, the aesthetic result is usually less than desirable.

ORTHO & TMJ:

Few orthodontists are aware of the many implications involved in moving the teeth. It is not enough to have the teeth line up nicely and look right. Their positioning has to be in harmony with the musculature and the temporo-mandibular joint.

Often teeth are moved without consideration for muscle balance, cranial alignment and the temporomandibular joint. This is a dangerous practice since all the joints of the head must be in harmonious relationship with one another for optimal health. The entire craniosacral system can be tremendously impacted by even a slight alteration in the positioning of the teeth.

IDENTICAL TWINS:

I began studying functional orthodontics because I wanted my patients to have a higher standard of care than was available with traditional orthodontics. At a seminar I attended, Dr. John Witzig presented a remarkable case study dramatically illustrating the disruptive effects of orthodontia. He showed us pictures of identical twins born in England. When they were teenagers, the parents took the twins to a public dentist under the socialized medical system, who recommended extracting the first bicuspids and fitting appliances for both children. They proceeded with one twin, but then had reservations and took the second twin

Often teeth are moved without consideration for muscle balance, cranial alignment and the temporomandibular joint. This is a dangerous practice since all the joints of the head must be in harmonious relationship with one another for optimal health.

to a private dentist who fitted appliances without extractions.

Dr. Witzig then displayed pictures of the sisters as adults several years after the procedures had been completed. When those photos went up, the audience literally gasped. *The two sisters were no longer identical.* The differences in their facial structure were striking. One sister had a beautiful broad smile and full balanced facial development. The other sister had a very narrow face and tight, unpleasant smile. Of course, you can guess that the sister with the unattractive facial features was the unfortunate twin who had her bicuspids removed.

TRADITIONAL VS. FUNCTIONAL ORTHODONTICS:

I cannot overstate the importance of the teeth in terms of proper bone development in the face and jaw. With traditional orthodontics, frequently teeth are extracted to make more room and then pressure is applied to move the remaining teeth around until they create proper bite and look straight. Unfortunately, very little attention is given to the effect of the procedure on the overall bone structure and musculature, and often the appearance.

However, there are some orthodontists who practice what is now being termed "functional orthodontics." In the above example, a functional orthodontist would evaluate the entire structure of the head, the relationship of the teeth to the jaw and other facial bones, and then fit an appliance that would stimulate growth and encourage teeth to realign themselves in proper relationship to the rest of the head and muscles. The entire mode of treatment, including the physical structure of the actual appliances, is different. Because a harmony is achieved between the muscles, and lip and tongue pressure, the chance of a relapse is greatly diminished.

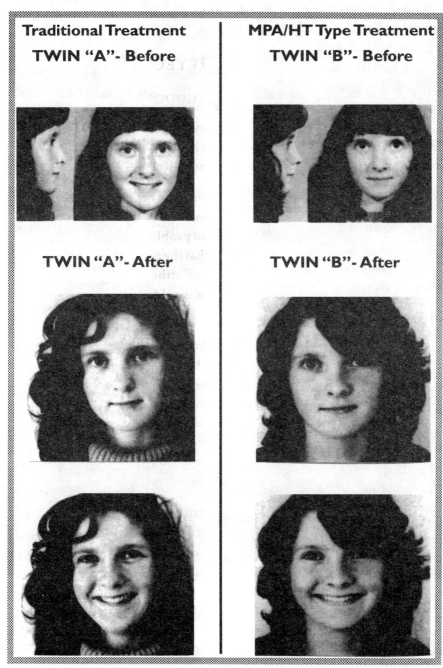

Figure 18.1 Identical Twins with Different Orthodontic Treatment

DENTAL DETECTIVE STORY

PAIN FROM ORTHODONTIC TREATMENT

A 35-year-old osteopathic physician called because she was having strange pains in her head, her body and her feet; backaches; discomfort in the TMD area and all manners of inexplicable physical problems.

A year before, an orthodontist had removed all four of her bicuspids and fitted her for an appliance to move her front teeth back and to realign her bite. I suggested her present problems were coming from her new bite - a result of the changes that the orthodontist made. She was upset because when she called the orthodontist to inquire, he told her that the alignment of her jaws would not cause any of these problems, including TMD.

I immediately referred her to an excellent orthodontist who appreciates the principles of Whole Body Dentistry. He corrected the changes which had caused her pain - compensating for the missing bicuspids, which never should have been removed. Shortly thereafter her pains and symptoms vanished. She was thrilled with the results, but there was one small remaining problem: one of her canine teeth would not go into proper alignment. The orthodontist tried everything, but the tooth stubbornly remained slightly out of position.

She and I had discussed amalgam removal in the past, and since the new orthodontic work was so successful, she decided to go ahead and have the amalgams removed. She was in the reception lobby paying her bill *when she literally felt the tooth moving in her head.* The stubborn canine tooth had simply and suddenly turned and righted itself! She was amazed - and so was I. The next day her chiropractor examined her and said that for the first time in years, her head, neck and body were all in perfect alignment.

NICKEL

There are other hazards associated with orthodontics. Most appliances are made out of stainless steel, which is nickel-based. There are major problems with nickel. At least 10% of all women are allergic to nickel. If your ears get irritated by earring posts, then most likely you fall into this category - and your body would be in a constant state of reaction to nickel-based orthodontics.

If your child is sickly or has allergies, you need to be especially diligent about compatibility testing. Fortunately, most children are very resilient and can withstand some insult to their systems. At a minimum you should be alerted to the side effects of dental materials, so that if a reaction occurs you will notice it right away. As mentioned above, these effects may intensify if there are mercury fillings present. Even if you are not allergic, the battery effect and electrical current generated by the stainless steel metal in the mouth (*see chapter 7*) can possibly create health problems.

ACUPUNCTURE MERIDIANS

Yet another factor to consider with orthodontics is the relationship of the teeth to the body's acupuncture meridians. As the teeth are repositioned, their relationship to the meridians is being impacted. We are barely beginning to understand what kind of long-term effect might occur from this type of interference with the meridians.

TREATMENT DECISIONS

Understand, I am not condemning orthodontics or extractions. When done properly the positive effects of orthodontic treatment with respect to the temporomandibular joint, cranial sutures, and self esteem are highly beneficial. If you are considering orthodontics for yourself or your children, simply realize that you need to make certain that your orthodontist comprehends the implications and actively factors them into the treatment plan.

It is also essential that you be aware of all possible reactions and early warning signs of problems. Some of these indicators

DENTAL DETECTIVE STORY
TMD FROM ORTHODONTIC TREATMENT

Dana was seven years old when I met her. Concerned about her receding chin, I checked the muscular tension in her jaw and face and confirmed that her orthodontic treatment was causing her to develop TMD. Her father was very upset with this news and insisted that her orthodontist was "one of the best." Several years later, with Dana's chin still receding and a bump developing on her nose, he relented and agreed to see an orthodontist I recommended for a second opinion. He confirmed that there were problems with her present braces.

Upset with the cost involved in having new braces made, the father returned to the original orthodontist who assured him that the braces were OK and his daughter would be fine. Six months later Dana developed severe ear aches. Her pediatrician said she had TMD. They went back to my recommended orthodontist, who removed the old braces and fitted her with appropriate functional appliances. Almost immediately her earaches stopped. Within three months her chin regained prominence and the bump in her nose straightened itself out.

might be quite subtle, some not as subtle. Chronic colds, lethargy, or irritability may appear. Facial changes that are unesthetic may occur. These must not be overlooked or bigger problems may develop.

As with all dental procedures, arm yourself with information and listen to your own best judgement.

CHAPTER 19

PEDODONTICS

Pedodontics is the dental specialty which treats children. Children begin getting their first teeth at about six months of age, and they have a full complement of "baby" teeth - dentists call them "deciduous" teeth - usually by the age of three. By about the age of six the child will begin losing the "baby" teeth as the permanent teeth come in. The last deciduous teeth are lost anywhere from 11 to 14 years of age.

Pedodontists treat children from infancy to the point when the child goes off to college. Particularly the early years of this period are extremely important. A child is constantly in the process of development; every day sees new changes. Every stage builds on the previous stages of development. Thus anything that has adverse effects on a child runs the risk of having impact on the rest of their life.

TOXIC INTRUSIONS:

Children's physical systems can be more vital and reactive than those of adults, so toxic intrusions can cause severe problems. Be extremely cautious of dental work with your children. Too many dentists recommend invasive dental procedures that can be devastating.

Dental Detective Story

A CHILD'S ILLNESS FROM DENTAL MATERIAL

A patient of mine told me about the terrible health problems her young son Evan was encountering. He would get so sick every few weeks that he would be unable to walk and had to be hospitalized. The doctors at Yale Medical Center were able to isolate that there was something wrong with his immune system, but they did not know what. I immediately asked her if any dental work had recently been done. Sure enough, a pedodontist had placed amalgams and stainless steel (nickel) crowns. I explained to her my suspicions and she brought him in right away. We took out the metals and he recovered immediately. In the fourteen years since this happened he has never had a recurrence of this problem.

We are usually completely unaware of the impact of this kind of dental work on young children. Since we do not recognize the problem, we do not have statistics to understand the scope of the issue. We have no way of knowing how many children may have suffered unnecessary illness brought on by dental procedures. Avoid taking a chance with your children's health.

STAINLESS STEEL CROWNS

Dentists, especially pedodontists, like to use stainless steel crowns on baby teeth. They can place these crowns rapidly, and insurance coverage is better than for amalgam. The problem is that a child can react to the nickel and become very ill, and no one will think that the illness comes from the child's dental work.

FLUORIDE

In addition to stainless steel crowns and amalgams, topical fluoride treatments can be dangerous for your child. I would also not recommend giving your child fluoridated water or fluoride tablets (*see chapter 20*).

DENTAL DETECTIVE STORY
A CHILD'S ILLNESS FROM DENTAL MATERIAL

When Tiffany was three, the pedodontist recommended and placed amalgam fillings and stainless steel crowns. Immediately following the procedure, this previously healthy, active toddler fell ill and had a dramatic increase in her white cell count. They suspected leukemia and placed her in the care of an oncologist. She had not gained a pound in a full year, suffered from recurrent fevers, low energy and a diminished immune system. When she came to me, I recommended that she be tested immunologically for dental materials, and she was found to be reactive to mercury and nickel. We removed all the metals in her mouth and she is now fine. The so called "leukemia" was simply a normal physical reaction to being poisoned by metals that the small child's system simply could not handle. It was a tragedy that should never have begun.

AMALGAM FILLINGS

I would strongly recommend that only nonmetal restorative materials be used for your child's dental work. Never, ever allow a dentist to put an amalgam filling in your child's mouth.

In addition, my own advice would be that any amalgam fillings in your child's mouth be removed as soon as possible by a reputable, properly trained Whole Body Dentist (see the appendix). If your child is ill, do not allow a dentist who is not properly trained in health, nutrition, and the correct process for amalgam removal, do the removal - or the results could be disastrous.

FINAL THOUGHTS:

Most dentists I know are ethical, caring individuals. Many of them, however, simply do not know the effects of some of their procedures. That is why as a patient, you need to recognize how dramatic and dangerous dentistry can be when it comes to your children.

CHAPTER 20

THE FLUORIDE PHENOMENON

Tここ here are many standard procedures and common practices promoted by the American Dental Association and taught in dental schools that have a generally unrecognized negative aspect. The use of fluoride is one of the most extreme and disturbing examples.

Everyone knows that "fluoride helps prevent cavities" because we have all heard it a thousand times from ADA endorsed toothpaste advertising campaigns. Many municipalities even fluoridate their drinking water. However, there is just one little thing about fluoride that is not being mentioned - it is extremely toxic.

Fluoride is a poison, and there is enough of it in one standard tube of toothpaste to kill a 20-pound child. It is a waste product of the aluminum and fertilizer industry; when it is introduced into a living body, it acts as an enzyme inhibitor that stops cellular functioning. Fluoride is, and has always been, listed as a lethal poison in the Merck Manual, the standard manual on diseases and toxins used as a reference by all physicians. Moreover, you can corroborate that information in virtually any toxicology reference book, such as Goodman and Gilman's **The Pharmacological Basis of Therapeutics**, the most renowned textbook of toxicology.

Adding insults to injury, worldwide studies have proven that adding fluoride to your drinking water is not at all effective in reducing or preventing tooth decay. Topical use of toothpaste or mouthwash probably is of some benefit because it will kill bacteria. After all, it is a rodentcide and insecticide. However, I feel there are safer ways to kill bacteria in the mouth.

Besides, caries (tooth decay) is primarily a systemic disease. Proper nutrition and balancing of body chemistry are the ultimate way to prevent decay. Dr. Price vividly demonstrated this in his book **Nutrition and Physical Degeneration**.

WHISTLE BLOWER:

Why is a known poison allowed in our drinking water and toothpaste? Dr. William Marcus, senior toxicologist in the Office of Drinking Water at the EPA, would like you to know the answer to that question. In 1990, Dr. Marcus, publicly denounced fluoride and "blew the whistle" on a cover-up of higher rates of cancer, birth defects, osteoporosis and especially hip fractures, in areas where water is fluoridated.

In particular, Dr. Marcus publicly questioned the honesty of a long-awaited government animal study designed to determine if fluoride causes cancer. Upon examining the raw data of the experiment, Dr. Marcus found clear evidence that fluoride causes cancer, and suggested that a review panel set up by the government to review the data had deliberately downgraded the results.

Dr. Marcus was promptly fired. Fortunately he sued, and in 1992 Administrative Law Judge David A. Clark, Jr. ordered the EPA to give him back his job, with back pay, legal expenses and $50,000 in damages.

The EPA - the agency which is supposed to protect the public from environmental risks - appealed. However, the appeal was turned down in 1994.

Among other things, it turned out that the EPA had shredded important evidence that would have supported Dr. Marcus in court. The original trial proceedings also show that EPA employees who wanted to testify on behalf of Dr. Marcus were threatened by their own management. EPA officials also forged some of his time cards, and then accused him of misusing his official time.

EFFECTS:

TOOTH DECAY

The original support for fluoride came in the late 1940's when a study conducted on rats indicated that fluoride might have an impact on tooth decay. A five-year, two-city study was conducted in which one city's drinking water was fluoridated and the other "control" city's water was unchanged. *During the five years of the study, there was a 65% decrease in tooth decay in BOTH cities.* However, the test results from the control city were not reported, so it would look as though fluoride had a miraculous impact on reducing decay. At the time, the Department of Health, Education and Welfare accepted the false test results and the fluoride phenomenon was off and running.

CONSUMPTION MISCALCULATIONS

Fluoride has become so prevalent in America's drinking water today that it is found in virtually all bottled beverages, including reconstituted juice. And because there were gross miscalculations in the amount of water people drink, many Americans in areas with fluoridated drinking water are consuming fluoride at levels that no one predicted. You would be horrified to learn that there are even documented cases of children actually dying in dental offices from swallowing fluoride while having topical fluoride applications to the teeth. Despite all this, dental students are still being taught that anyone who opposes the use of fluoride in drinking water is a fanatic and is harming the public.

"MOTTLED" TEETH

One of the most obvious signs of a child's excessive exposure to fluoride is the "mottling" of teeth. Dentists will sometimes tell you that white spots on your teeth are related to fevers when

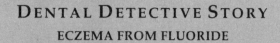

DENTAL DETECTIVE STORY
ECZEMA FROM FLUORIDE

A mother brought her five-year-old son to my office for a dental exam. His face was covered with persistent eczema. She had tried food elimination and various other informal treatments, both medical and non medical. I asked her about fluoride in the child's water and toothpaste. The water in their community was fluoridated, and the child had been using fluoridated toothpaste.

I suggested that she give the child bottled water and use non fluoridated toothpaste. In a few weeks, the mother called to say that her son's skin was now clear.

you were young. Not so; usually these chalky white areas on teeth are the result of fluorosis, which in its more advanced stages can cause discoloration, pits and crevices, and in general, weaker teeth - not stronger ones.

While the American Dental Association does admit that white spots on teeth are linked to fluoride, they consider them a minor cosmetic problem. The truth is that fluoride actually changes the cellular structure of the tooth enamel in the formative years when the tooth is developing.

Studies done at the University of Rochester showed that 28% of children aged 11 to 13 living in areas with fluoridated drinking water had fluorosis. What else might it also be affecting? Isn't it naive to think that fluoride is only affecting the formation of teeth and nothing else?

OTHER SIDE EFFECTS:

Even the ingestion of a very small amount of fluoride can cause significant side effects.[16]

Taking one-half to one milligram of fluoride per day - the quantity of fluoride found in one to two pints of fluoridated water - may result in the following symptoms:

■ black, tar-like stools	■ bloody vomit	■ diarrhea
■ stomach cramps or pain	■ nausea	■ faintness
■ tremors	■ weakness	■ constipation
■ loss of appetite	■ pain and aching of bones	■ stiffness
■ sores in the mouth	■ unusual increase in saliva	■ eczema
■ weight loss	■ white, black or brown discoloration of teeth	

FLUORIDE CAUSES AGING

Those of us who do not exhibit any of these overt symptoms will have a form of subclinical deterioration we commonly call "aging".

Fluoride speeds up the aging process by inhibiting the production of enzymes which are essential to supply certain chemical reactions in the body. It also breaks down collagen, the main supportive protein of skin, tendon, bone, cartilage, connective tissue and, of course, teeth. Genetic damage and disruption of the immune system have also been linked to fluoride because it interacts with and distorts the forces which maintain the normal shapes of different body proteins.

The resulting effect is that the immune system attacks its own protein. We are seeing increasing numbers of these so-called "auto-immune" diseases in recent years.

IMPACT ON WHITE BLOOD CELLS

Small amounts of fluoride can cause significant bodily upset. For example, at the levels found in fluoridated drinking water, fluoride will enter the bloodstream causing a decreased migration of white blood cells. This renders these essential bacteria-fighting agents less able to travel through the blood to where they are needed. It has also been shown that the presence of fluoride in the blood stream decreases the ability of the white blood cells to "phagocytize," or destroy, bacteria and other foreign agents. Another effect of ingesting fluoridated water is a decreasing level of thyroid activity.

STUDIES:

OSTEOPOROSIS

Fluoride is highly invasive to the human system and interferes with basic cell growth and functioning. In 1978, Yale University researchers Dr. J. A. Albright and colleagues reported at the American Orthopedics Research Society that exposure to as little as one ppm (parts per million) of fluoride decreases bone strength and elasticity, leading to osteoporosis.[17] Water can be legally fluoridated with up to four parts per million - although only one ppm is recommended. A report from the National Institute of Arthritis and Metabolic Diseases published in 1973 reported that there was a 50 to 100% increase in the occurrence of osteitis fibrosa in patients whose artificial kidney machines were run with fluoridated water.[18]

DNA REPAIR ENZYME

In 1974, the Austrian physician Dr. Wolfgang Klein reported that as little as 1 ppm of fluoride inhibits the essential DNA repair enzyme by 50% causing chromosomal damage.[19] This DNA repair enzyme slowly decreases during the natural aging process, which is why there is an increase of birth defects in babies born to women over the age of 40. But if fluoridation is destroying the DNA repair enzyme in young women, the result could be increasing birth defects at much younger ages. There are numerous medical studies demonstrating the link between small amounts of fluoride and genetic damage. There is a strong link to cancer as well.

CANCER

Dr. Dean Burk, former Chief Chemist Emeritus at the U. S. Cancer Institute, and Dr. John Yiamouyiannis in a 1977 study, compared the cancer death rates of the 10 largest non-fluoridated cities and the 10 largest fluoridated cities to their original pre-fluoridation cancer death rates from 1940 through 1950. They discovered that in the fluoridated cities, from 1952 (when fluoridation began) to 1969 there was a 10% fluoride related increase of cancer deaths. There was no comparable increase in the non-fluoridated cities during that same period of time. The largest increases occurred primarily in people ages 45-64 and in people 65 and over.

Fluoride has become so prevalent in our drinking water, bottled beverages, reconstituted juices, that many Americans are consuming fluoride at levels no one predicted.

IQ

In recent studies on rats exposed to sodium fluoride, it is shown that the central nervous system is affected - and that affects on behavior depend on the age at exposure. [20]

In China studies on children indicate a lowering of IQ. In a study of 907 children aged 8-13 years, it was demonstrated that IQ was related to the amount of fluorosis. In areas of moderate to severe fluorosis, they surmised that the central nervous system was affected during fetal development or early infancy thus affecting intelligence.[21]

DURATION AND DOSE:

How serious is the threat of fluoride poisoning for you and your family? Well, let's start with toothpaste. The average 7 oz. tube has approximately 100 ppm fluoride - that is enough to kill a

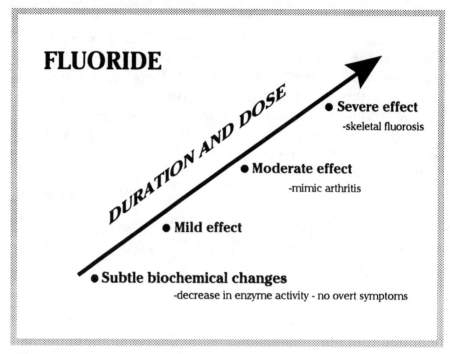

Figure 20.1 Fluoride - Duration and Dose

twenty pound child if the entire tube were consumed. If toothpaste were subject to the same labeling laws as household cleansers, manufacturers would be required to inform you that it is a toxic substance and should be kept out of reach of children!

Like mercury, we are dealing with an exposure to small amounts of a toxin over a long period of time. This makes it difficult to establish a relationship and offer a proper diagnosis. We must always *remember the combined effect of duration and dose.* It is interesting that when the EPA set its standard for lead in the air, they argued that to prevent more serious effects, they needed to limit the more subtle biochemical changes that lead was provoking in children. However, with fluoride, if crippling skeletal fluorosis is not present, the EPA deems all other degrees of fluoride-induced changes irrelevant. I also wonder about the combined effects of mercury and fluoride. We know that mercury impairs renal function, and as renal function declines, systemic levels of fluoride increase. Also pipe corrosion increases by as much as 100% with fluoridated water. This leads to increased levels of lead and copper.

We are all ingesting fluoride in unspecified dosages from a number of sources. Like mercury, we are dealing with an exposure to small amounts over a long period of time. We must always remember the combined effect of duration and dose.

BECOME AWARE

Fluoride is a problem, and we are all ingesting it in unspecified dosages from a number of sources. What can you do to avoid fluoride? The first step is to become aware. Call your local water authority and find out if your drinking water is fluoridated. If it is, try to organize a city or town referendum to change it. However, the power and propaganda of the ADA is such that even a referendum against fluoridating the water is not always enough. A patient of mine related how her town had a referendum that voted against fluoridating the water supply. Through various mechanations, those that thought they knew what was best for the voters, had the water fluoridated.

OTHER SOURCES

Remember, most home filters will not eliminate fluoride, so you may need to use bottled water. Carefully check the labels to ensure you do not buy fluoridated spring water. Avoid using fluoridated water to cook rice, pasta, hot cereals, beans, soups, or to brew tea and coffee.

It can be difficult to find a good toothpaste and mouthwash that does not contain fluoride at the local supermarket. You will most likely need to visit a health food store. You also need to read labels avidly since some orange juices, beers, and soy milks have fluoride, if made with fluoridated water. Buy 100% juices, not reconstituted ones, and check baby food labels to see whether they are reconstituted too. Most water in commercial use is fluoridated. If possible, try to find out whether the fruits and vegetables you purchase have been fertilized with fluoride-contaminated phosphates.

Another precaution is to ask your family dentist not to use topical fluoride treatments. I think that "Do you use topical fluoride?", should be one of the first questions you ask before deciding to visit a new dentist.

FINAL THOUGHTS:

There is no doubt in my mind that the entire issue of fluoride is a political one. The scientific studies clearly show fluoride's dangerous effects. What is most shocking is that there are no conclusive studies showing that fluoride added to the drinking water does indeed decrease tooth decay. The addition of fluoride to drinking water is highly irresponsible. If you feel as outraged as I do about this, I encourage you to express your concern to legislators and health care leaders. Dr. John Yiamouyiannis' book on fluoride is an excellent book on the history, politics and effects of flouride *(See Appendix)*.

PART IV

TOOLS OF THE TRADE

CHAPTER 21

ELECTRO-ACUPUNCTURE ACCORDING TO VOLL (ELECTRO-DERMAL SCREENING)

Whole-Body Dentistry incorporates the use of adjunct "alternative" treatment methods to assist in healing, balance the massive effects of dentistry, and reduce symptoms as well as to create a favorable human environment for healing. A good Biological Dentist will be familiar with all of these methods. At a minimum, your dentist definitely should be working in close conjunction with thoroughly trained professionals in each of these methods, so that alternative therapies can be utilized to improve your treatment and speed your healing process.

ELECTRO-DERMAL SCREENING:

Nearly everyone has heard of an MRI these days. Consider that up until a few years ago, the average person had *never* heard of it - and you will begin to get an appreciation for how quickly technology is advancing to support our application of energetic medicine. One such advance has been with Electro-acupuncture According to Voll (EAV), which is also sometimes called Electro Dermal Screening (EDS). Your dentist may not have heard of it yet, but this piece of equipment will undoubtedly be as common as the dental chair and X-ray machine in several years.

This amazing instrument will revolutionize the way that dentistry and medicine are practiced in the next century. The

At the minimum, your dentist should be working in close conjunction with thoroughly trained professionals, so that alternative therapies can be utilized to improve your treatment and speed your healing process.

technology is based on the phenomenon (which you should now be familiar with) that all parts of the body are interrelated and are also energetically linked via meridians.

HOW DOES IT WORK?

EAV was developed out of the research of Dr. Reinhold Voll, an M.D., anatomy professor, and acupuncturist, who began his clinical analysis in the late 1940's. Dr. Voll was able to scientifically document something that Chinese acupuncture had known for centuries. In the human body, there are higher levels of electrical conduction - or in other words, areas of less resistance - at certain points on the skin, many of which correspond to traditional acupuncture points. Fascinated by this, he developed a simple metering device to measure the skin resistance on acupuncture points. The meter had a metal cylinder at one end and a stylus at the other.

Dr. Voll would have his patient hold a small brass cylinder in one hand. He would then touch the tip of the stylus to a specific acupuncture point. The cylinder would introduce a minute amount of electrical current, which would travel through the body to reach the stylus, thus forming a complete electrical circuit. The amount of skin resistance at the acupuncture site would then be recorded. Dr. Voll found that normal skin resistance over a healthy point is 100,000 Ohms. This equals 50 on the Voll Galvanic Skin Response Scale. During 40 years of research, Dr. Voll actually documented an entire network of energetic pathways throughout the body, better known as energy meridians. Many corresponded to traditional acupuncture meridians; many are new. He was also able to establish that each meridian acted like a "highway" for energy, connecting specific teeth, organs, tissues - in fact, everything in the body.

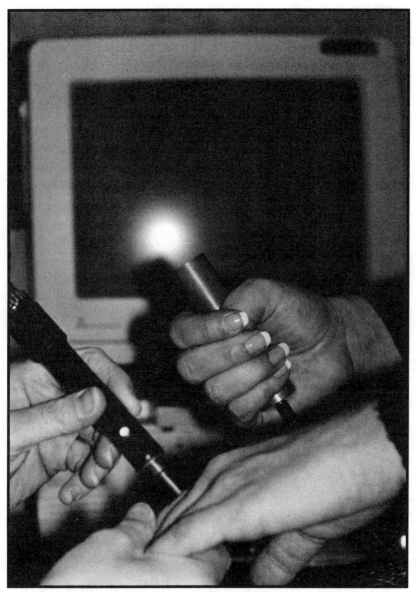

Figure 21.1 Photograph of EAV Screening

The major part of the EAV equipment is basically an Ohm meter, measuring electron flow in a circuit. The body operates largely by a series of electrical impulses which have been shown to follow certain pathways. We access these pathways via points on the skin where there are changes in the electrical resistance or the ability of the tissue to conduct electricity. A healthy pathway will be able to sustain a certain level of electron flow. Inflammation tends to foster increased activity in the cells, with all sorts of chemical reactions going on, creating a more active environment through which electrons can flow at a greater rate. Thus, if inflammation exists anywhere along the pathway, the EAV will show a higher than average flow of electrons, and a reading greater than 50 will be indicated.

Degenerative states cause cellular activity to slow and stagnate, making it more difficult for electrons to flow through the circuit, with a reading of less that 50 being indicated. The most significant information from EAV testing occurs when the circuit has a high electron flow, which then drops to a lower reading. This indicates that a circuit which was formerly capable of sustaining an electron flow, is no longer able to do so and usually evidences a disturbance in the circuit. The result is a reading which drops. Dr. Voll called this fall in reading an "Indicator Drop."

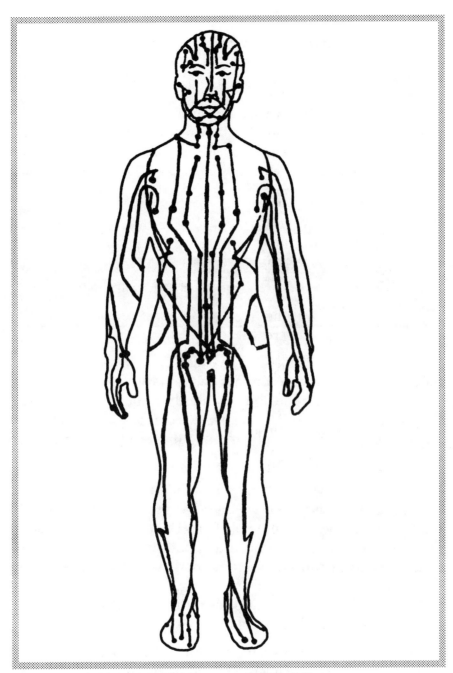

Figure 21.2 Diagram of Acupuncture Meridians

DENTAL DETECTIVE STORY
BONE INFLAMMATION

Linda, age 43, came into my office with a very sore upper right molar. She said it felt like the tooth was being pushed out and the pain radiated over the right side of her head. She had no decay, no gum problems, and a clean X-ray, yet the tooth was sensitive to tapping and mimicked a tooth needing root canal. With Electro-Dermal Screening, I discovered a disturbance in the intestine meridian. I checked the tooth area associated with that meridian and discovered a chronic low-grade inflammation in the bone behind the aching tooth. Cleaning out the bone brought immediate relief. Without the "tools" of energetic medicine, Linda would have most likely gone ahead with a root canal and come out of it still in pain.

Because the body consists of an energetic "web" of relationships, the major circuits have secondary and tertiary circuits connecting virtually all parts of the body. A highly skilled practitioner of EAV testing can establish a cause-effect relationship between any two points on the body, making it a vastly powerful tool.

MERIDIAN LINKS

Since every major organ and, in fact, nearly everything in the human body is linked via meridians to a specific tooth, the implications of the EAV in Whole-Body Dentistry are tremendous. For instance, EAV may indicate a hypothyroid condition which could actually be caused by a root canal in the upper first molar. This could provide an early warning, after which traditional testing could be performed to see if the condition has reached a point where blood tests are reactive.

In my own practice, I have encountered repeated instances where inflammation or energetic "problems" with the tonsil area have been accompanied by knee problems. And I have had two young diabetic patients, both of whom experienced the onset of their disease following trouble with their tonsils and wisdom teeth. The idea that there may be a relationship between these events would baffle, and perhaps elicit derision, from a Western-trained physician, yet it is completely consistent with so much of the progress in energetic medicine.

INVESTIGATIONAL DEVICE:

Although used in Europe for medical diagnosis, EAV is still considered an investigational device in the United States. But that does not mean it cannot be employed as an aid to support diagnosis. EAV is currently being explored by the FDA as a noninvasive diagnostic instrument. A phenomenal amount of information is available through EAV testing, about the nature of what is happening in the body. It is an exceptional tool for helping to recognize what types of more traditional diagnostic testing might be appropriate to confirm suspicions of what is occurring.

This equipment has also been used for allergy testing and one study has actually shown EAV to be as accurate, or MORE accurate, than other forms of allergy testing.[22] Studies are being done in this country to show the value of this type of testing in screening for diabetes.

In my practice, I find EAV testing may make me aware of possible jaw bone infections, and then I can use other diagnostic methods to confirm. And I often use EAV and an awareness of energy meridians to test my suspicion that two seemingly unrelated symptoms in the body are indeed linked.

ENERGETIC STRESSORS:

Electro-Dermal screening can provide invaluable information on the patient's energetic "web" or currents and help determine the location of "energetic stressors" which create blockages or disturbances in the natural flow of energy. The stressors themselves

THE TEETH AND THE BODY
ENERGETIC INTER-RELATIONS

American Academy of Biological Dentistry
P.O. Box 856, Carmel Valley, CA 93924, 408-659-5385

Chart — Upper arch (maxilla), read left → right; ‖ = midline

ENDOCRINE GLANDS: PITUITARY GLAND ANTERIOR LOBE · PARA-THYROID · THYROID · THYMUS · POSTERIOR LOBE · INTERMEDIATE LOBE (PITUITARY GLAND) · PINEAL GLAND ‖ PINEAL GLAND · POSTERIOR LOBE · INTERMEDIATE LOBE (PITUITARY GLAND) · THYMUS · THYROID · PARA-THYROID · PITUITARY GLAND ANTERIOR LOBE

SENSORY ORGANS: INTERNAL EAR / TONGUE · TONGUE · NOSE · EYE, POSTERIOR PORTION · NOSE ‖ NOSE · EYE, POSTERIOR PORTION · NOSE · TONGUE · INTERNAL EAR / TONGUE

PARANASAL SINUSES: MAXILLARY SINUS · ETHMOIDAL CELLS · SPHENOIDAL SINUS / FRONTAL SINUS ‖ SPHENOIDAL SINUS / FRONTAL SINUS · ETHMOIDAL CELLS · MAXILLARY SINUS

JOINTS: SHOULDER, ULNAR SIDE / ELBOW, ULNAR SIDE / HAND, ULNAR SIDE / FOOT, PLANTAR SIDE TOES / SACRO-ILIAC JOINT · JAW / ANTERIOR HIP ANTERIOR KNEE MEDIAL ANKLE JOINT · SHOULDER, RADIAL SIDE / ELBOW, RADIAL SIDE / HAND, RADIAL SIDE / FOOT, BIG TOE · POSTERIOR KNEE / HIP / SACROCOCCYGEAL JOINT / ANKLE JOINT / LATERAL · POSTERIOR ‖ POSTERIOR KNEE / SACROCOCCYGEAL JOINT / HIP / ANKLE JOINT / POSTERIOR · LATERAL · SHOULDER, RADIAL SIDE / ELBOW, RADIAL SIDE / HAND, RADIAL SIDE / FOOT, BIG TOE · JAW / ANTERIOR HIP ANTERIOR KNEE MEDIAL ANKLE JOINT · SHOULDER, RADIAL SIDE / ELBOW, RADIAL SIDE / HAND, RADIAL SIDE / FOOT, PLANTAR SIDE TOES / SACRO-ILIAC JOINT

SEGMENTS OF THE SPINAL MARROW AND DERMATOMES: SC 2 SC 1 / STH 1 SC 8 / STH 7 · STH 6 · STH 5 / SS 2 SS 1 · SC 2 SC 1 / STH 12 STH 11 / SL 1 · SC 2 SC 1 / SC 5 SC 6 SC 7 / STH 2 · STH 3 · STH 4 / SL 4 SL 5 · SC 2 SC 1 / STH 8 / STH 9 / STH 10 · SC 2 SC 1 / SL 3 SL 2 / SS 5 SS 4 SS 3 / SCo ‖ SC 1 SC 2 / SL2 SL3 / SS 3 SS4 SS 5 / SCo · SC 1 SC 2 / STH 8 / STH 9 / STH 10 · SC 1 SC 2 / SC 5 SC 6 SC 7 / STH 2 STH 3 STH 4 / SL 4 SL 5 · SC 1 SC 2 / STH 11 STH 12 / SL 1 · SC 1 SC 2 / SC 8 / STH 1 STH 5 / STH 6 STH 7 / SS 1 SS 2

VERTEBRAE: C 2 C 1 / TH 1 C 7 / TH 7 · TH 6 · TH 5 / S 2 S 1 · C 2 C 1 / TH 12 TH 11 / L 1 · C 2 C 1 / C 7 C 6 C 5 / TH 4 · TH 3 · TH 2 / L 4 · L 5 · C 2 C 1 / TH 8 / TH 9 / TH 10 · C 2 C 1 / L 3 L 2 / S 5 S 4 S 3 / SCo ‖ C 1 C 2 / L 2 L 3 / S 3 S 4 S 5 / SCo · C 1 C 2 / TH 8 / TH 9 / TH 10 · C 1 C 2 / C 5 C 6 C 7 / TH 3 TH 4 TH 2 / L 4 L 5 · C 1 C 2 / TH 11 TH 12 / L 1 · C 1 C 2 / C 7 TH 1 / TH 5 TH 6 TH 7 / S 1 S 2

ORGANS: HEART RIGHT SIDE — DUODENUM RIGHT SIDE TERMINAL ILEUM · PANCREAS — OESOPHAGUS STOMACH RIGHT SIDE · LUNG, RIGHT SIDE — LARGE INTESTINE, RIGHT SIDE · LIVER RIGHT SIDE — GALL BLADDER BILIARY DUCTS RIGHT SIDE · KIDNEY, RIGHT SIDE — URINARY BLADDER RIGHT SIDE GENITO-URINARY AREA RECTUM ANAL CANAL ‖ KIDNEY LEFT SIDE — URINARY BLADDER LEFT SIDE GENITO-URINARY AREA RECTUM ANAL CANAL · LIVER, LEFT SIDE — BILIARY DUCTS, LEFT SIDE · LUNG, LEFT SIDE — LARGE INTESTINE, LEFT SIDE · PANCREAS — OESOPHAGUS STOMACH, LEFT SIDE · HEART LEFT SIDE — DUODENUM LEFT SIDE JEJUNUM ILEUM

TISSUE SYSTEMS: CENTRAL NERVOUS SYSTEM / LIMBIC SYSTEM ‖ CENTRAL NERVOUS SYSTEM / LIMBIC SYSTEM

OTHER SYSTEMS: MAMMARY GLAND RIGHT SIDE ‖ MAMMARY GLAND, LEFT SIDE

TEETH DIAGRAM: RIGHT RETRO MOLAR SPACE MAXILLA ‖ LEFT RETRO MOLAR SPACE MAXILLA

American and European Nomenclatures:

1	2	3	4	5	6	7	8	9	10	11	12	13	14	15	16
18	17	16	15	14	13	12	11	21	22	23	24	25	26	27	28

32	31	30	29	28	27	26	25	24	23	22	21	20	19	18	17
48	47	46	45	44	43	42	41	31	32	33	34	35	36	37	38

TEETH DIAGRAM: RIGHT RETRO MOLAR SPACE MANDIBULE ‖ LEFT RETRO MOLAR SPACE MANDIBULE

Chart — Lower arch (mandible), read left → right; ‖ = midline

OTHER SYSTEMS: ENERGY EXCHANGE · MAMMARY GLAND RIGHT SIDE ‖ MAMMARY GLAND, LEFT SIDE · ENERGY EXCHANGE

TISSUE SYSTEMS: PERIPHERAL NERVES · ARTERIES VEINS · LYMPH VESSELS ‖ LYMPH VESSELS · VEINS · ARTERIES · PERIPHERAL NERVES

ORGANS: TERMINAL ILEUM / ILEO-CECAL AREA — HEART RIGHT SIDE · LARGE INTESTINE RIGHT SIDE — PANCREAS · OESOPHAGUS STOMACH, RIGHT SIDE PYLORUS PYLORIC ANTRUM — LUNG, RIGHT SIDE · GALL-BLADDER BILIARY DUCTS, RIGHT SIDE — LIVER, RIGHT SIDE · RECTUM ANAL CANAL URINARY BLADDER RIGHT SIDE GENITO-URINARY AREA — KIDNEY, RIGHT SIDE ‖ RECTUM ANAL CANAL URINARY BLADDER LEFT SIDE GENITO-URINARY AREA — KIDNEY, LEFT SIDE · BILIARY DUCTS LEFT SIDE — LIVER, LEFT SIDE · OESOPHAGUS STOMACH, LEFT SIDE — LUNG LEFT SIDE · LARGE INTESTINE LEFT SIDE — SPLEEN · JEJUNUM ILEUM, LEFT SIDE — HEART LEFT SIDE

VERTEBRAE: C 2 C 1 TH 1 / C 7 TH 7 TH 6 TH 5 / S 2 S 1 · C 5 C 6 C 7 / TH 2 TH 3 TH 4 / L 4 L 5 · TH 12 TH 11 / L 1 · C 2 C 1 / TH 8 / TH 9 / TH 10 · C 2 C 1 / L 3 L 2 / S 5 S 4 S 3 / Co ‖ C 1 C 2 / L 2 L 3 / S 3 S 4 S 5 / Co · C 1 C 2 / TH 8 / TH 9 / TH 10 · TH 11 TH 12 / L 1 · C 5 C 6 C 7 / TH 2 TH 3 TH 4 / L 4 L 5 · C 2 C 1 TH 1 / C 7 TH 7 TH 6 TH 5 / S 1 S 2

SEGMENTS OF THE SPINAL MARROW AND DERMATOMES: SC 2 SC 1 / STH 1 SC 8 / STH 7 STH 6 STH 5 / SS 2 SS 1 · SC 2 SC 1 / SC 5 SC 6 SC 7 / STH 2 STH 3 STH 4 · SC 2 SC 1 / STH 12 STH 11 / SL 1 · SC 2 SC 1 / STH 8 / STH 9 / STH 10 · SC 2 SC 1 / SL 3 L 2 / SS 5 SS 4 SS 3 / SCo ‖ SC 1 SC 2 / SL 2 SL 3 / SS 3 SS 4 SS 5 / SCo · SC 1 SC 2 / STH 8 / STH 9 / STH 10 · SC 1 SC 2 / STH 11 STH 12 / SL 1 · SC 1 SC 2 / SC 5 SC 6 SC 7 / STH 2 STH 3 STH 4 / SL 4 SL 5 · SC 1 SC 2 / SC 8 / STH 1 STH 5 / STH 6 STH 7 / SS 1 SS 2

JOINTS: SHOULDER-ELBOW, RIGHT SIDE / HAND, ULNAR SIDE FOOT, PLANTAR SIDE TOES / SACRO-ILIAC JOINT · HAND, RADIAL SIDE FOOT BIG TOE · ANTERIOR HIP ANTERIOR KNEE / MEDIAL ANKLE JOINT / JAW · HIP · POSTERIOR KNEE / SACRO-COCCYGEAL JOINT / ANKLE JOINT / LATERAL · POSTERIOR ‖ POSTERIOR KNEE / SACRO-COCCYGEAL JOINT / ANKLE JOINT / POSTERIOR · LATERAL · HIP · MEDIAL ANKLE JOINT / ANTERIOR HIP ANTERIOR KNEE / JAW · HAND, RADIAL SIDE FOOT BIG TOE · SHOULDER-ELBOW, LEFT SIDE / HAND, ULNAR SIDE FOOT, PLANTAR SIDE TOES / SACRO-ILIAC JOINT

PARANASAL SINUSES: ETHMOID CELLS · MAXILLARY SINUS · FRONTAL SINUS / SPHENOIDAL SINUS ‖ FRONTAL SINUS / SPHENOIDAL SINUS · MAXILLARY SINUS · ETHMOID CELLS

SENSORY ORGANS: MIDDLE EXTERNAL EAR TONGUE · NOSE · TONGUE · EYE ANTERIOR PORTION · NOSE ‖ NOSE · EYE ANTERIOR PORTION · TONGUE · NOSE · MIDDLE EXTERNAL EAR TONGUE

ENDOCRINE GLANDS: GONAD · ADRENAL GLAND ‖ ADRENAL GLAND · GONAD

Figure 21.3 EAV chart of teeth and organs

can be anything alien or out of balance in the body, including fillings, crowns, impacted teeth, root canal teeth, sinuses, tonsils, scars, out-of-alignment teeth, impacted teeth, inflamed gums and improperly healed extraction sites. Even scars located on different parts of the body can act as stressors affecting important meridians.

Stressors create a field of disturbance in the energetic web of the body. These fields of disturbance are most often in the head, because the mouth is where we most readily allow thoughtless or unnecessary surgery, excessive procedures, and implantation of foreign materials. The results of the disturbance can be felt anywhere in the body and can virtually block any treatment's effectiveness.

Every individual has his or her own tolerance level for stressors. Some people walk into my office with a mouth full of metal, yet their systems have adjusted and handled the impact admirably. Yet another patient could have just one amalgam filling and be suffering from devastating illness. It is really incredible what a range of response there is to stressors. Certainly factors like diet, exercise, state-of-mind, genetics, and general well being play an important role. Continued research in stressor and energetic disturbances is essential and the EAV is an invaluable tool for this purpose.

DR. VOLL'S BREAKTHROUGH DISCOVERY:

Ironically, a mishap at a presentation of EAV technology by its originator resulted in the discovery of one of its most powerful abilities. Dr. Voll was giving a demonstration of an EAV device on a patient who had a large "Indicator Drop" on his prostate point. During a break, a helpful homeopath from the audience approached the patient and offered him a remedy. The patient gratefully put the vial of medication in his pocket. After the break,

A highly skilled practitioner of EAV testing can establish a cause-effect relationship between any two points on the body, making it a vastly powerful tool.

Dr. Voll resumed the demonstration with the same patient; yet he was baffled because the readings on the prostate point were now normal.

After several confusing and somewhat embarrassing minutes of questioning his subject to figure out what was going on, he discovered the homeopath's remedy. Although the remedy was in a container in the patient's pocket, it was able to influence the readings. In fact, they discovered it influenced the readings when it was simply held near enough to be in the subject's energy field. When removed beyond the patient's energy field, the reading again indicated inflammation of the prostate.

This event, which could have resulted in the defamation of Dr. Voll's research, ultimately led to one of the most interesting discoveries surrounding meridians. It also created a spectacular demonstration of how the human energy field does indeed extend beyond the boundaries of the physical body. In the following years, Dr. Voll continued to work with homeopathic remedies and developed a very sophisticated, yet highly effective, means to select proper homeopathic remedies based on EAV readings.

Dr. Voll placed a tray in circuit between his EAV machine and the patient. He could then place homeopathic remedies, vitamins, foods, or anything else on this tray, to test their effects on the meridian reading. Dr. Voll was also able to test the effects of different potencies. Surrounding him would be thousands of test items. Today, the new EAV units are computerized and are called "Electro Dermal Screening" devices. Designers of these units have figured out how to incorporate the energy signature of the various homeopathic remedies, supplements, foods, drugs, etc., into the software, so that bottles of the actual matter being tested are not necessary. Via the computer, all the various potencies *(see chapter 27)* can be tested. Everything is then stored to disk.

COMPUTERIZED REMEDIES:

Another exciting breakthrough involving these Electro-dermal Screening devices is that the energetic signal from the computer can be imprinted into a bottle of water, yielding a potentized remedy. I was very skeptical that a remedy made in this manner could be effective, and for a long time, did not use remedies made in this fashion. Then two things happened that changed my mind.

The first was that one of my patients presented on an emergency basis with severe pain on the left side of her face. Five days earlier, I had removed a tooth from the upper left jaw, and until that day she had no problems. This is a classical sign of "dry socket". However, upon EAV testing, a dry socket was not indicated. Upon reflection I decided to see if the remedy for inflammation of the parotid salivary gland would balance the EAV reading. Voila! It did. The patient, not knowing what I was doing, was left with the silent balancing energetic signal being broadcast while I took a phone call. When I left, she was holding her face, rocking in pain. Upon my return, about five minutes later, she was smiling and pain-free. She said, "I don't know what's going on, but I'm fine now."

I made a dose of that energetic signal for her to take that night upon retiring, and she never had the problem again. It was an enlightening experience. However, I still was not 100% convinced that making a remedy from this electronic signal could be effective - at least until the next incident.

I was playing softball and had a severe collision with another ballplayer. In the accident I was knocked out momentarily, having broken a few ribs and having sustained a heavy blow to the mouth. A very high dosage of the homeopathic remedy Arnica did wonders

DENTAL DETECTIVE STORY
WISDOM TEETH

Anne Marie first came into my office wearing an oxygen mask. Several years earlier she had been exposed to chemicals used for furnace cleaning. The entire family got sick, but Anne Marie continued a downward slide. When I met her, she was so ill that the slightest exposure to any airborne chemical, however minor, would cause an extreme reaction. She was unable to drive, used an oxygen mask almost continuously and was rapidly getting worse. We removed her mercury fillings which stopped her downward slide and even resulted in some very slight improvement, but she was still extremely ill. I ran EAV tests on her and discovered that her wisdom teeth were energetically affecting her autonomic nervous system and allergy point. She also had severe periodontal problems around these teeth, and consequently I urged her to have them removed. She resisted and continued under the care of an environmental physician, but saw little improvement.

Over the next two years I repeated the testing and consistently determined that the wisdom teeth were energetically related to her other problems. Finally she agreed to have them removed. When she returned for her next visit she gleefully informed me that not only had she driven herself on the 200-mile trip to my office, but that she was down to less than one canister of oxygen a week, from her average of five! According to Anne Marie, the results of the procedure were instantaneous, "like someone turning on a light switch" and that immediately following the extractions her heart rate, which previously had been greatly elevated, had returned to normal.

for my extremely swollen lip and my chest pain. However, one of my lower front teeth became very sensitive to any temperature change, even to the air as I talked. Injection of different homeopathics adjacent to the tooth did not help.

After a month, I realized I was probably facing a decision on having a root canal or extracting the tooth. At this time I was attending an EAV seminar. I asked one of the instructors to find a balancing energetic signal for the sensitive tooth. He imprinted the corrective signal at appropriate potency into a glass of water and I took a sip. About four hours later, I was eating some cold fruit and suddenly realized that I no longer had any pain! That was three years ago; I have had no problems since that time.

"LIKE CURES LIKE":

A fundamental principal of homeopathy is that *"like cures like."* Knowing this, Dr. Voll reasoned that if homeopathic mercury, for example, will balance a previously unbalanced point, then mercury must be at least a part of the problem on that meridian. These concepts seem quite elusive because they are based on the principles of energy rather than the mechanical model which is more familiar.

Using the principle of "like cures like," a physician specializing in oncology, Dr. Vincent Speckhart, is doing remarkable research with cancer using the EAV. He introduces pathology slides with different types of cancer into the "field" of a cancer patient until he finds the slide that balances, thereby determining what type of cancer may be present. This is then checked against biopsy reports. Dr. Speckhart is also able to determine the optimal dose of chemotherapy needed, usually finding the amount necessary to be much less than the quantity traditionally used. He is amassing a tremendous amount of data and has come to realize the significant relationship between cancer and dental stressors.

CHAPTER 22

KINESIOLOGY

Kinesiology as a Whole-Body Dentist would use it involves what is called "muscle-testing." A muscle's resistance to a slow build-up of force will be measured and then will be re-measured as something is placed into the patient's energy field.

For instance, if a patient holds their arm straight out to the side and I press down on the wrist with a slow build-up of force, at a certain point the patient's arm will no longer be able to resist. The applied pressure and the point at which the muscle can no longer resist can be measured objectively with instrumentation, or subjectively by the person testing. Clinical Kinesiology testing is almost always done subjectively. This works very well because if something detrimental to the patient is introduced into the patient's energy field, for example by giving it to the patient to hold, a previously strong muscle will exhibit definite weakness. A good kinesiology tester can gain a lot of valuable information in a short period of time. I use some kinesiology testing as part of my initial exam.

HEAVY METAL TOXICITY SCREENING:

Dr. Dietrich Klinghardt, a prominent physician and teacher of neural therapy and kinesiology, taught me a method to screen for heavy metal toxicity, especially mercury, using muscle testing. By placing the center of my palm over the patient's umbilicus (belly button), a previously strong muscle should go weak. If it does not, I have the patient hold a vial of DMPS, a strong chelator of mercury. If the muscle then goes weak while my hand is over the umbilicus, then I know that mercury is a problem for that patient. I can say that because of having seen a positive correlation of the umbilicus test with hundreds of EAV and provoked urine test results. The umbilicus test is also a fast way to monitor a patient's progress as they undergo chelation therapy after mercury removal.

If something detrimental is introduced into the patient's energy field, a previously strong muscle will exhibit definite weakness. A good kinesiology tester can gain a lot of valuable information in a short period of time.

OTHER DENTAL USES:

I also find kinesiology very useful at the dental chair. If a patient has a tooth hurting, but does not know which one, and upon examination I can not find anything, I will test kinesiologically. I will have the patient therapy-localize, meaning I have them touch a tooth and see if a strong muscle goes weak. I will have them touch each tooth in the area until I get a weak reading. That will be the offending tooth.

I remember one patient who insisted her pain was in the upper right molar area. All the teeth tested fine kinesiologically, until I got to her front tooth. She insisted the pain could not be coming from that area. I placed a little anesthetic above the front tooth, and the pain disappeared. I find this technique to be extremely accurate.

In short, kinesiology is a very valuable tool when used in conjunction with other dental diagnostic methods.

CHAPTER 23

NEURAL THERAPY

Neural Therapy was fortuitously discovered by the German physicians Ferdinand and Walter Huneke in 1925, as a result of one of those accidents of clinical treatment which have advanced medicine so much over the centuries.

The Huneke brothers had a sister who suffered from severe migraines. For years with great frustration, they could not find anything to provide relief. An older colleague had told Ferdinand about a remedy which he had found helpful for the pain of rheumatism. During one of his sister's violent attacks, he decided to try an intravenous injection of the substance. While injecting, miraculously the violent pain disappeared, along with the dizziness and nausea that accompany a classic migraine. Needless to say, after so many failures, they were elated.

Interestingly, the headaches did not reoccur. What was this miraculous product? The remedy came in two forms: one for intravenous injection without Procaine (Novocaine) and a version with Procaine for painless muscular injection. Dr. Ferdinand Huneke accidentally used the second form, intravenously. Upon further investigation, it was discovered that it was the Procaine that was responsible for the unexpected cure. Prior to this it was thought that Procaine used intravenously would cause death, so it was fortunate that he accidently injected the Procaine compound.

DENTAL DETECTIVE STORY
NEURAL THERAPY

Georgia (about 42) came to me for a dental examination. She had good dental health, some amalgams and one root canal of her upper left bicuspid. In taking her history, one of the things that she related was constant abdominal pain of three years duration. Gynecological examinations and other examinations by physicians proved negative. What I did was to inject some anesthetic around the root canal tooth. Very often this will act to block the signal from a focus (which is a localized reaction having effects remote from that site) and give us an idea of what it might be affecting.

During energetic testing I had been able to relate the root canal tooth to the large intestine - the bicuspid is on the lung/large intestine meridian. So as not to influence the patient, I did not tell her why I was injecting above this tooth. However, I left her alone for a few minutes, and when I came back, she said, "What did you do? My abdominal pain is gone!"

Repeating the procedure on a following visit, with the same results, she decided to remove that root canal tooth, and in the past five years has had no reoccurrence of the abdominal pain.

NEURAL PATHWAYS FOR A CURE:

In 1928, the brothers published the results of their clinical experiments using Procaine under the title, "Unfamiliar Remote Effects of Local Anesthetics." They showed that the effect was on the nervous system, not via the blood stream, by obtaining relief through local injections. The healing process was faster than the Procaine could be absorbed. Only the autonomic nervous system could give results with such speed. Hence the term, "Neural Therapy" -the use of neural pathways for a cure.

The autonomic nervous system controls the automatic functions of the body: breathing, heartbeat, digestion, hormone production, metabolism, etc. It is the upset of this autonomic regulatory system which leads to disease. Injection of Procaine helps reestablish the proper electrical balance in the nerves and tissues, thereby balancing the autonomic regulation.

The heart of this regulatory system is in the fluid and tissue that surrounds every cell, called the interstitial tissue. It is here that the nerve endings of the autonomic nervous system, the blood vessels and the lymph system all come together. This is where all the vital functions are ultimately controlled, and this is the center of regulation or dysregulation. It is via this interstitial fluid that every cell in the body communicates with every other cell in the body. Because of this, a scar, an inflammatory reaction, a foreign body, a dead tooth, etc. can create a disturbance which has local or distant effects. Procaine can help balance this dysregulation.

Neural Therapy is comprised of two types of treatment. One is called segmental therapy. This was the basis of treatment for the first sixteen years of the Huneke brothers' neural therapy practice. Segmental therapy consists of procaine injections directly into the problem area, which often exhibit pain or itching. Upon repeated injection, the balance in the interstitial tissues returns and the symptoms disappear. For instance, specific injections into the area of the prostate are often of great benefit in resolving an enlarged prostate gland.

Discovery of the second type of neural therapy occurred by accident. Dr. Ferdinand Huneke was treating a patient for a painful frozen shoulder. Thinking to deaden the pain, he injected Procaine directly into the shoulder. The next day the patient returned and told Huneke that while her shoulder was still frozen, an old scar on her leg had become extremely itchy. Huneke then gave the

DENTAL DETECTIVE STORY

WISDOM TEETH

Mary's feet went numb when she turned 63; the numbness remained for seven long years. Now, at 70, she had all but given up hope. Every so often she would try a new doctor, but none could solve the puzzle. Neurological workups, CAT scans, and all kinds of tests revealed nothing. Then she came across a Naturopathic physician who told her that he thought the problem might be in her mouth.

The first thing I noticed on Mary's Panoramic X-ray were her impacted wisdom teeth. Since that area of the mouth relates to the peripheral nerves, I thought it might be causing the problem. I tested this theory with Neural Therapy - to create a change in the electrical potential of this area. I injected a drop of procaine over each wisdom tooth. Sensation in the soles of her feet came back immediately. She was stunned, and immediately decided to have the wisdom teeth removed.

patient a second Procaine injection - directly into the itchy scar (presumably to deaden the itching effect). To the astonishment of both doctor and patient, after the injection into the scar, the patient instantly regained full and complete motion in her shoulder.

This near instantaneous result has been given the name "lightening reaction," and the area of underlying dysregulation is termed an "interference field." This interference field creates an aberrant signal which goes out over the cellular web via the interstitial tissue, and instantly resonates with an area that is injured or inherently weak. As long as the transmitter and receiver resonate this inharmonious signal, symptoms will manifest. An injection into the transmitter (i.e., the scar) will shut off the signal and give relief to the receiver (i.e., the shoulder).

WHOLE BODY DENTISTRY & NEURAL THERAPY:

Through observation of these connections, neural therapy has clearly proven the link between the mouth and other parts of the body. Whole Body Dentistry often incorporates the principals of neural therapy to help demonstrate which oral transmissions may be having distant effects. The Hunekes found the most prominent disturbance field to be the tonsils, root canals or diseased teeth, and scars.

Neural Therapy is a marvelous diagnostic tool, especially effective if a patient needs to decide whether a particular procedure is truly going to have the benefits the doctor suspects it will. I have used it time and time again to help my patients understand how problems in their body are related to their mouth. Neural Therapy bears an obviously close relationship to EAV and other types of energetic healing therapies.

CHAPTER 24

LASERS

Laser is an acronym for Light Amplification by Stimulated Emission of Radiation. Laser light is produced by using electricity or intense light to excite what is called the active medium. This medium can be a solid, liquid, gas, or semiconductor. The power output is measured in watts and can be in the form of a constant or pulsed wave. Also unique to laser light versus regular light are the properties of coherence, monochromaticity and unidirectionality. Monochromatic means that there is only one specific wave length, and coherence means that all the energy waves are in phase. Unidirectionality allows the laser beam to remain concentrated even over a great distance.

"HOT" LASERS:

Today everyone is familiar with laser light shows, lasers for eye surgery, and lasers for removing spider veins in the legs. Lasers are also used in dentistry for periodontal surgery and for vaporizing tooth decay. These devices are "hot" lasers and have a high energy output. They are relatively new and will become more and more a part of everyday medicine and dentistry.

"COLD" LASER:

Another type of laser is known as a "cold" laser. Here the output of energy is much lower so that thermal damage cannot occur. Use of these low output devices has resulted in Low Level Laser Therapy (LLLT) which is widely used throughout the world. Research has shown LLLT to be beneficial for:1) stimulation of cell growth (except for cancer cells); 2) overall increase in tissue activity; 3) edema reduction; 4) anti-inflammatory effects; 5) acute and chronic pain relief. The wavelength found to be most beneficial in most instances is 830 nanometers.

"MODIFIED" LASERS:

Use of LLLT is not legal in the United States as of yet. Research is ongoing and approval by the FDA is hopefully near. While waiting to be able to purchase a laser, I purchased a 30 milliwatt light of 830 nanometers that was not a true laser because it was not coherent, meaning one could look at the light and not cause eye damage. Interestingly, I have found the same results as with LLLT. Therefore, I surmise that it is the wavelength which is of utmost importance followed by the power. One must have at least 30 milliwatts of power to have any penetration into bone. Consequently, when I personally speak of using LLLT, I am referring to this "modified" laser.

ACUPUNCTURE POINTS

Using LLLT on acupuncture points is very beneficial. I have seen good results placing the lights on different sinus points relieving a sinus headache. One can also treat a specific acupuncture point and verify a change with EAV. This is helpful in identifying what else is affected by that point. After balancing, i.e. the tooth point, you can check the previously abnormal i.e. heart point and see if that now has been balanced, thus indicating an interrelationship.

DENTAL USES

One published study detailed the healing of cavitations with LLLT and the subsequent clinical health improvement.[23]

Using LLLT after oral surgery seems to be of benefit in helping post-op pain and swelling.

One area where the laser has hardly ever failed is in the treatment of teeth that are sensitive due to the recession of the gum. This causes the root to be exposed often with painful consequences, especially to cold air or water. Placing the laser against the root for one minute almost always gives immediate relief to temperature change.

Low Level Laser Therapy is another useful tool of the trade.

CHAPTER 25

NUTRITION

O f the 125 Medical Schools in the U.S., only 32 have a required course in nutrition for graduating physicians. This dismal situation is even worse in dental education programs. There is a very strong perception that diet and nutrition are unrelated to the teeth - but this could not be farther from the truth.

Many people now realize that they must be responsible for figuring out for themselves just what is proper nutrition. But, these days there are so many conflicting viewpoints that it is hard to decide what constitutes healthy eating. Every ten years it seems the so-called experts flip-flop their position and tell us to eat exactly what they told us not to eat before. First butter is bad and margarine is good; then butter is good and margarine is bad. What do you do?

DR. WESTON PRICE:

I have followed the field of nutrition closely for more than 20 years, and what I have discovered is that there are a few very good, very consistent individuals in the field whose work and advice has consistently held up under scrutiny over time. Dr. Weston Price was a giant in this field. In his book, **Nutrition and Physical Degeneration**, long considered the seminal text on nutrition, he documents the effect of dietary changes on bone structure, teeth and health in general.

In his extensive travels to Alaska, the Amazon, Australia, Europe, the South Pacific and many other areas, Dr. Price consistently found that those people who remained on their native diets experienced almost no tooth decay or periodontal disease, and that degenerative diseases in general were virtually non-existent. However, when the "white man's" civilized diet, including refined sugar and flour, was introduced, tooth decay and other degenerative diseases began appearing with sudden and alarming frequency. Perhaps the most dramatic proof of the link between diet and health was demonstrated by Dr. Price through these studies.

There is a very strong perception that diet and nutrition are unrelated to the teeth - but this could not be farther from the truth.

Dr. Price also noted that the new diet brought about remarkable changes in physiognomy. Bodies actually became narrower and taller. The dental arches became narrower, causing tooth crowding. Womens' pelves also became narrower, making childbirth more difficult.

One photo essay of two brothers indisputably illustrated these changes. The first brother stayed on the family farm and continued to consume the traditional native diet. The second brother had moved to the city and switched to a typical modern diet. The brother on the farm had no tooth decay whatsoever, while the city brother had now developed rampant decay. What is truly remarkable, though, is that when the city brother moved back to the farm and resumed his native eating habits, all decay ceased.

Based on Dr. Price's research, following a genetically appropriate diet would lead to optimal health. This does not make for highly practical advice, however, as native genetic lines are for the most part completely blurred. Most of us do not live in isolated tribal communities, marrying into our own genetic pool. How then do we apply Dr. Price's insights to our modern dietary needs?

CALCIUM & PHOSPHOROUS:

The studies of Dr. Price and subsequently Dr. Melvin Page showed an important indicator of health to be the calcium and phosphorous values of a fasting blood report. Calcium and phosphorous bind in a ratio of approximately 2.5:1, with optimal fasting blood readings of 10 mg/dl of calcium, to 4 mg/dl of phosphorous. As calcium increases relative to the phosphorous, beyond the 2.5:1 ratio, free calcium increases. Anything that depresses phosphorous will produce more free calcium. This is where diet and nutrition come in. By following a certain diet and then drawing blood, and observing the resulting effects on your calcium and phosphorous levels, we can determine what diet is genetically optimal for the individual.

The things that especially depress phosphorous are sugar - particularly refined sugar; caffeine; and alcohol. Depending on the individual, one glass of wine may have a tremendous negative influence on the phosphorous; while for another person it may take three glasses of wine.

FIVE BASIC DEFECTS

On a daily basis, it is not practical to draw blood. Another way to observe the effect of our food on our bodies is to monitor salivary pH. The same foods that tend to depress phosphorous will cause a lowering of the salivary pH, which indicates a more acid body. A vicious cycle is set in motion, leading to the five basic defects common to all degenerative diseases:

1. **Acidemia:** your system is more acid.

2. **More free excess calcium**: as acidemia increases, free excess calcium rises.

3. As free calcium rises, **uncontrolled chronic inflammation** appears.

4. Uncontrolled chronic inflammation leads to **connective**

tissue breakdown.

5. **Oxidative stress**, resulting from free radical production[24]

The increase in free radicals leads to greater acidemia, thus perpetuating the cycle. Any oxidative catalyst, like pesticides or heavy metals, will further perpetuate this cycle.

According to Sam Queen, an expert in this area of nutrition, all degenerative diseases have these five defects in common, and it is critically important to begin treatment by correcting the acidemia as the first step. Removal of the oxidant catalyst first - for example, removing amalgams - prior to correcting the acidemia and free calcium excess, will place further oxidative stress on the system, often leading to a worsening of symptoms.

MAINTAINING YOUR PH BALANCE:

There are a lot of nutritional clues in the mouth which are discovered during the examination. For example, a big buildup of tartar in the mouth can indicate an imbalance of calcium metabolism. This is a very common condition and is far more serious than you might think. An imbalance in the calcium metabolism tends to indicate that pH is out of the optimal range in the body. PH reflects the acid-alkaline balance of your body.

CALCIUM

It is important to really understand what occurs in your body when your calcium is too high or too low. As you know, calcium is the primary mineral of bone. Almost all the calcium in your body is in your bones. A tiny percentage - only 1%, actually - is found in your blood plasma and fluids. Out of that 1% that is not in your bones, about half of it is unbound and is called free calcium. The free calcium floats around your system in an unbound state, looking for something to pair up with.

Free calcium is tremendously important and is vital in initiating a lot of healthy metabolic functions. These calcium molecules can be found on the cell membranes. Periodically they burst through microscopic channels into the cells, creating a reaction which allows the cells to function properly.

A very minuscule amount of calcium creates these essential positive reactions; that is why even a small reduction in the amount of calcium in your body could actually have a powerful effect on the health of your overall system. And if the reverse occurs, and you have an excess of free calcium, then instead of periodic bursts, the calcium will continuously and repeatedly burst into the cells. This increased frequency will cause problems, just as a deficiency does. Heart medications known as calcium channel blockers are designed to help manage this problem, but it could also be resolved by bringing the free calcium levels on line by balancing the pH through diet and supplementation.

ACID PH & INTESTINAL PROBLEMS

People with acid pH often begin to experience problems digesting certain foods. This occurs because the intestine becomes inflamed and permeable to the passage of proteins. When large proteins pass through the walls of the intestines in this manner, the body realizes that they do not belong there and will react to them as though they are foreign matter. This in turn sets up allergic reactions to certain foods. A propensity to yeast infections can also occur with these types of intestinal problems because "candida" - a fungus normally present in a healthy intestine - also gets out of balance. Combine an acid pH with mercury and the problem is compounded. It is astounding how many mercury toxic patients have intestinal problems and thus food allergies, and candida.

MERCURY AND THE GUT

Antibiotic resistance and the rise of "superbugs" receive a lot of press today. The spectre of becoming ill with a rampant infection and not having an effective antibiotic available is not a pleasant thought.

Research by Dr. Anne Summers at the University of Georgia in collaboration with Drs. Lorscheider and Vimy at the University of Calgary Medical School demonstrated that when monkeys had amalgam fillings placed, their intestinal bacteria developed substantial mercury resistance.[25] Most significant was the resistance these same bacteria developed to two or more antibiotics. Certainly this is not the only cause of antibiotic resistance; however it is one we can avoid.

Mercury is now being linked to the rising levels of antibiotic resistance.

ORAL PH IMBALANCE

As a dentist, when I look into someone's mouth, one of the first things I consider is my patient's pH balance. If there is evidence of periodontal disease, a lot of plaque or calculus, caries, loose teeth, or receding gums, I immediately know there is a pH imbalance resulting in free calcium.

Oral pH should be at least 6.5, and preferably right around 7. When pH levels get below 5.5, the body will actually begin demineralizing bone and enamel to try to regain the balance it needs. This is the start of tooth decay. The jaw and teeth are one of the first places the body will do this, and it is also the first sign of osteoporosis.

The jawbone is just the first location of the disease. If steps are not taken to stem the disease, it will migrate from the jaw to other bones. Most dentists would interpret periodontal disease as primarily related to bacteria in the oral cavity. When you consider that bacteria thrive in a warm, moist, sweet and acidic environment - an acidic mouth is basically heaven to bacteria.

However, in periodontal disease, the actual underlying cause is not linked to bacteria. It is systemic, and generally linked to the five defects common to all degenerative diseases listed above.

Periodontal disease should also be considered the first step leading to full-blown osteoporosis. It is very important that dentists begin to understand this phenomenon.

RAISING YOUR pH:

To raise your pH, here is what you do:

1. Cut out refined sugars and concentrated natural sugars (for example, oranges and bananas have more concentrated sugars than apples.) Keep fruit juices to a minimum; if you must have juice, drink small amounts of apple juice.

2. Eliminate caffeine and alcohol.

3. Increase your intake of cultured dairy products, like plain yogurt or cottage cheese. Do NOT eat hard cheeses. In addition to raising pH, cultured dairy products keep unfriendly bacteria in check in the intestines.

4. Include other cultured foods like sauerkraut or soy products - they are good too.

5. Fresh squeezed lemon juice in water is excellent for bringing up pH.

Bringing the body back into a healthy balance this way will also give you stronger recuperative power.

DIETARY CHANGES

In addition to evaluating pH, I often recommend other specific dietary changes, especially during the process of amalgam removal. Also, proper attention to diet just before, during and after surgical procedures, can help the body fight infection and hasten the healing process -- even minimizing the need for pain medication.

Often one of my recommendations is that my patients eat

eggs, because the sulfur in eggs is superb at bonding with excess metals and toxins and carrying them out of the system. Of course, nearly everyone is shocked at the suggestion of eating a lot of eggs because of all the attention to low cholesterol diets.

CHOLESTEROL:

Cholesterol is an area where there is a lot of information and a lot of misinformation. You probably did not know that studies have shown a higher incidence of cancers, especially colon cancer, in individuals with cholesterol levels below 160. Yet the medical standard today is to get cholesterol down as far as possible, rather than the more optimal level of around 200-220.[26]

Cholesterol-lowering drugs have been advertised as reducing the death rate due to heart disease. Statistically speaking, that is true. But what you have not been told is that *the death rate from all causes is the same or higher when people are on the cholesterol lowering drugs*. As with anything else, a little bit of moderation is in order when trying to manage your cholesterol levels. You never want to rapidly and dramatically alter the balance of anything in your body - including cholesterol.

It seems as if high levels of cholesterol are sometimes an appropriate response to excess heavy metals in the body, if for example you have amalgam fillings. It is hypothesized that excess cholesterol is sometimes the body's way of managing the influx of toxins from mercury fillings. If you unwittingly interfere with the cholesterol levels you may experience extremely serious effects from the unmanaged metals in your system.

This seems to be the situation of a friend of mine who is also a dentist. Several years ago he decided to get *really* healthy. He read all the latest nutrition books, went on a strict macrobiotic diet, and got his cholesterol way down. Shortly thereafter he developed Parkinson's Disease. A homeopathic physician examined him and told him that he had a classic case of mercury poisoning, probably caused by handling a lot of mercury in his dental practice. His "high cholesterol" probably had been buffering the mercury in his body.

My friend refused to accept that diagnosis and is unwilling to listen to information from me either. Sadly, to this day he will not consider treating his progressing illness as mercury-related.

Essentially, though, the responsibility for good nutrition rests on the patient. I can review the blood work, evaluate the information revealed by examination, and make recommendations. I always explain the effects of nutrition and the specific dietary factors most essential to each individual person's recovery. But I cannot go home with my patients and make sure they are eating well. Fortunately, most of my patients are usually eager to make the necessary changes in their eating habits, once they begin to understand the relationship between what they eat and their overall health.

SUPPLEMENTATION:

Before beginning treatment, especially on a sick patient, I will work on balancing his or her chemistry. Certain types of health questionnaires, hair analysis, blood analysis, and EAV will help determine what supplements to give. In addition, homeopathic tissue salts and remedies - specific ionic minerals and herbs - may also be utilized.

NATURAL VS. SYNTHETIC

In giving supplements, an important consideration becomes Natural vs. Synthetic. Picture this: A bottle of Vitamin C, and an orange. One is man-made, and one is God-made. Which is better?

Over the years my philosophy with reference to supplements

(vitamins and minerals) has evolved into a realization that natural is better. Supplements in their natural configuration are different from separated parts of nutrients. Taking a supplement that is fractionated may at times be necessary and beneficial, but in my opinion we must realize we are using it as a drug. As Dr. Royal Lee, a world-renowned nutritionist said, "A refined vitamin (synthetic or isolated) is as unsound as refined sugar."

The goal of all health treatments is to place the body in homeostasis. That is the point at which all bodily functions are working optimally and have the ability to return to this optimal point after being stressed. Think of it as an elastic band, stretched between your thumb and forefinger. If you pull and stretch one side and let go, the elastic band will return to its original shape. In a sense, it will return to homeostasis. If the elastic is brittle, however, when it is stretched it will break.

I believe that receiving vitamins and minerals in food form, as nature intended, is the best way to achieve this balanced state. Unfortunately, today it is hard to find foods which have the vitamin and mineral content of years ago, and therefore supplementation is often necessary.

Within the foods containing, let us say, Vitamin E, there is a broad biological complex which contains different forms of vitamin E - for example, Alpha and Gamma Tocopherol, and all the synergistic co-factors necessary for proper uptake and utilization, such as minerals and enzymes. However, when one normally buys Vitamin E, the label will read that it is only "Alpha Tocopherol." Or with Vitamin C, it will say, "Ascorbic Acid." These are only part of the vitamin complex. I favor a brand derived from organically grown foods, that has all the fractions present. The brand that I like is available only through licensed health care practitioners.

As with root canals, mercury and fluoride, I find that it is often beneficial to go back in time and explore an issue at the time of its initial debate. It is here before one side or the other has established itself as "victor" with all the entrenchment that follows, that we can often see the real truth.

In going back with reference to vitamins, study after study showed that in treatment of various maladies, isolation of fractions of different vitamin complexes did not yield the same results as did the whole complex. Studies showed that synthetic vitamins were not only inferior in effect, but in fact could be toxic and harmful - something a natural complex cannot be. A recent long-term study showed that men taking synthetic beta-carotene had an 18% higher incidence of lung cancer, more heart attacks, and an overall 8% higher death rate. Also, those taking Vitamin E had more strokes.[27]

The researchers were confounded, having believed that supplementation would have been beneficial. If only they had used a truly natural form of Vitamin A and E, I wonder what the outcome may have been. Remember, living things have an electromagnetic force surrounding them. This can be seen by Kirlian photography, and the display of this energy field is not the same in the synthetic variation.

Also, personal observation has led me to the conclusion that natural is better. I would see patients who were taking large amounts of supplements; true, they would often seem to feel a little better. However, upon EAV testing, they were not doing very well. Also, if they stopped taking the supplements, any benefits would reverse. I view this as a suppression of symptoms, just as with a drug.

Another question that has to be asked: with so many of our foods today being fortified with vitamins and minerals, why should anyone need additional supplementation? I believe the problem is that they are fortified with synthetic vitamins and minerals.

CHAPTER 26

HAIR ANALYSIS

I find hair analysis to be another useful tool, along with supplementation and diet recommendations. Hair analysis tests for minerals, and in general, I would say mineral imbalance is more important than vitamin levels. What is important on the hair analysis results are not so much the absolute values of the hair minerals, but the ratios. Of course, the absolute values cannot be far from optimal.

For instance, a normal ratio of calcium to magnesium in the hair is about seven parts calcium to one part magnesium. A very high ratio of calcium to magnesium, for example, 15 to 1 or greater, indicates a sensitivity to carbohydrates, and this person will benefit from a high-protein, low-carbohydrate diet. If the individual has not been on that kind of diet, they usually will feel much better if they cut down their consumption of carbohydrates. Another useful ratio is calcium to potassium. If the calcium to potassium ratio is greater than approximately five, it indicates an underactive thyroid; the greater the ratio, the weaker the thyroid.

I have also found that a very high hair calcium level usually indicates the patient will be slower in responding to treatment. The calcium is a form not readily utilizable and blocks normal function. In fact, these people are actually "starving" for calcium.

Hair analysis will also screen for heavy metals, and I have seen some high lead levels in both children and adults, which prompted referrals to an M.D. It seems that hair analysis is not particularly good for indicating a mercury problem, however. Many patients who have high mercury on urine testing may not have high hair mercury. If mercury is high in the hair, there definitely seems to be a problem.

CHAPTER 27

HOMEOPATHY

H omeopathy is a branch of medicine that has been in existence since the 1700's. It was created by the work of Dr. Samuel Hahnemann (1755-1834), an orthodox physician, and also a chemist, mineralogist and botanist.

It is a highly successful program of treatment with "remedies" that was extensively used by physicians in this country and around the world until the advent of penicillin. When this new "wonder drug" came into use, it was idealized as a preparation that would treat anything and everything. And in the years following introduction of antibiotics to medical practice, doctors ceased to employ the old remedies.

As the use of penicillin spread, homeopathy's popularity waned and the homeopathic medical colleges began to close. Unfortunately, because antibiotics were and still are taken far too frequently - and often for mild symptoms which could be readily cured by less dramatic means - people build up resistant bacterial strains or systemic familiarity and the antibiotics then cease to be effective. We are now in the age of "superbugs" that defy treatment, because of our indiscriminate use of antibiotics (and amalgams).

The drug companies are continually trying to come up with new and stronger strains of antibiotic medication. These constant research and development costs have dramatically increased the price of pharmaceuticals. The irony is that many of the symptoms currently being routinely treated with antibiotics could be more effectively alleviated with homeopathic remedies at a tiny fraction of the cost. And the remedies are non-toxic and less invasive to the human system.

I have already related how my wife and I personally became aware of homeopathy when our first-born son, Adam, had chronic ear infections for the first three years of his life, and was saved from having tubes surgically implanted in his ears by homeopathic treatment.

DENTAL IMPLICATIONS:

I started to wonder what other unnecessary and even dangerous procedures are regularly performed on people who could easily be cured by homeopathic remedies. I began to seriously consider some of the techniques I had been taught in dental school, and whether they were indeed the best course of care for my patients. I decided it was important for me to learn homeopathy as an adjunct to my dental practice.

Homeopathy is truly amazing. Without it, so many of my patients would have been forced into terrible treatment decisions. There are hundreds of stories like Anne's *(see page 192)*, of people with no remaining options being completely cured by homeopathic remedies. And while the use of homeopathy in dentistry is generally for acute situations, any good biological dentist should be versed in its capabilities for chronic use and work in close connection with a fully trained homeopathic specialist. One of the most often used benefits of homeopathic remedies has been in minimizing swelling and discomfort in post-operative patients. I never routinely use antibiotics after surgery, nor prescription pain medications. I find injection of homeopathic remedies to the surgery site, followed by oral homeopathic remedies and digestive pancreatic enzymes, is all that is required almost all of the time.

DISCOVERING "LIKE CURES LIKE":

Homeopathic Medicine has been espousing the mind-body connection for 200 years. In fact, the mental state of the patient is often the single most important diagnostic "clue" in finding the appropriate remedy. Especially with chronic disease, state-of-mind is the key symptom. Homeopathic treatment is based on the law of similars, and the principle that "like cures like." This means that substances which induce symptoms in a healthy person will cure those same symptoms in an ill person.

It is very interesting how Dr. Hahneman uncovered this law of nature. Upset with the side effects of the treatment of his time, Dr. Hahneman left practicing medicine. Being fluent in many languages, he translated medical texts from one language to another. In translating one article, he noticed that an overdose of the bark of the cinchona tree gave symptoms which he recognized were the same as those of malaria. He found this interesting, because cinchona bark was a treatment at that time for malaria. Dr. Hahneman then did a proving upon himself. He took repeated doses of the cinchona over several days, and came down with what would be called malaria. This led him to the idea that *like cures like*."

PROVINGS

Dr. Hahnemann then set out to do provings of other substances. He would take a group of healthy students, and would repeatedly give small amounts of a certain plant or other substances until symptoms were elicited. The students would record their mental, emotional and physical symptoms in a very systematic manner. Some of the symptoms would be common to all, and would be given more prominence: i.e., all would salivate profusely. Dr. Hahneman compiled the results of these provings in the **Materia Medica.** Knowing that in a healthy person, "X" would cause, for example, the left eye to twitch, and the left hand to become painful, Dr. Hahneman then knew that if a person came to him sick, complaining of a painful left hand and twitching left eye, the administration of "X" would take the symptoms away.

In fact, this is the same principle that the Salk vaccine and most modern immunological treatments are based upon: a virus that will induce an illness in its normal state can also induce immunity to the illness if given to the patient in a form that is weakened or dead.

*B*ecause the homeopathic remedy is working at an energetic level, the effect, especially in an acute situation, is often very rapid, but is at all times non-toxic and safe. If the wrong remedy is given, there will be no healing reaction, but also no harm to the patient.

DILUTIONS

With Homeopathy, however, the process by which the medicine is made is completely different. The effective healing agent, usually a plant, is soaked in alcohol. A drop of this tincture is then diluted one part to 99 parts distilled water. This is a 1C (one to one hundred). If diluted in ten parts of water, you have a 1X dilution. Then a method called "succussing" is employed to rapidly agitate the solution until the 1% agent is fractionally suspended throughout the solution. Then one part of this 1C dilution is placed in another 99 parts of water, and again succussed. This yields a 2C (one to one thousand) dilution, and so on up.

This dilution procedure may be repeated many times, and this sequence of dilution and succussion is called *potentization*. The dilution arrived at, i.e., 6C, is called the potency. In chemistry it is thought, that if one has a dilution beyond 10^{24}, there will not be even a single molecule of the original substance present. A dilution of 12C or greater is at or beyond this point. It is here that orthodox thinkers balk. In medicine, the more one delivers of a drug, the more the effect. How can a substance that has been diluted beyond the point of having even a single molecule of the original substance have any effect? Yet curiously enough,

CHAPTER 28

FLOWER ESSENCES

Dr. Edward Bach was a very well-respected, conventional physician, specializing in bacteriology, who practiced in London in the early 1900's. Dr. Bach developed an interest in homeopathy, became a homeopathic physician, and ended up practicing homeopathic medicine exclusively. Through observation, he came to the conclusion that the mental and emotional symptoms are the key to physical cure.

Bach perceived the relationship of the mind to higher subtle energetic bodies and because of his extreme psychic sensitivities, was able to uncover the effects of flowers on the mental emotional plane.

In seeking a method to unlock the vibrational frequencies of the flowers without going through laborious homeopathic potentization, Bach found that if specific flowers were laid upon spring water in full sunlight for several hours, the vibrational frequency of those flowers would be imprinted upon the water. Dr. Bach developed 38 flower remedies, with a recording of their emotional and mental characteristics. Today the number of flower essences has been greatly expanded, with flowers from all over the world being used.

DENTAL USES:

I find using flower remedies another useful tool in helping the dental patient's overall energetic well-being. One of the remedies

the more diluted the solution, the more powerful the healing agent becomes, without the attendant side effects and toxicity.

I think of it as unleashing the atomic energy of the original substance. Research has shown that biological activities of substances can be transferred to water. What happens is that the water molecules change their shape ever so slightly, as they pick up the energetic signal of the original substance as the potentization procedure occurs. Thus, the subtle energetic signal of the homeopathic remedy affect, at a subtle energetic level, the person or animal receiving it. Remember, we are 99% water.

DISEASE RESONANCES:

Is this how the remedy works? No one knows for sure. Hypothetically, it would seem that the physical and etheric body will resonate at a certain frequency in a healthy state, and with disease will resonate at another. If one can cancel the disease resonance, which is imposed upon the normal resonance, health will be restored. A traditional homeopath will find the appropriate resonance or remedy by the total symptom picture, mental and physical, of the patient. A practitioner using EAV will electronically uncover the proper frequency. Because the remedy is working at an energetic level, the effect, especially in an acute situation, is often very rapid, but is at all times non-toxic and safe. If the wrong remedy is given, there will be no healing reaction, but also no harm to the patient.

DENTAL CHOICES:

I feel all my patients can benefit from homeopathic remedies while undergoing dental treatment. I will, however, also use modern drugs, or "allopathic" treatment, when appropriate. There are times when an antibiotic or pain medication may be the best option.

DENTAL DETECTIVE STORY

HOMEOPATHY

"Please take out these teeth, Dr. Breiner." Anne had tears in her eyes as she pointed to her upper right jaw. Pretty, young and pregnant, she was exhausted to her breaking point as she begged to have her teeth removed. The pain they were causing her was excruciating. She had not slept in days and her physician could not find any cause. He did not want to prescribe pain relievers because Anne was pregnant.

The dental exam revealed nothing; her condition was baffling. Then I looked up Anne's state of mind and pain symptoms in a homeopathic repertory (symptom book) to find a specific homeopathic remedy that matched Anne's symptom picture. Twenty minutes after her first dose, the pain was completely gone and never came back. Anne was free to return home to her two small children, pain-free, and with all her teeth.

I have noticed, though, that patients who regularly use non-toxic homeopathic methods generally need less of the pain medication for a much shorter period of time.

TREATMENT DECISIONS:

With the administration of drugs, as with all treatment decisions, it is essential for the patient to be aware of the implications of standard procedures and the alternatives. Homeopathy is a highly effective, very safe option that has been overlooked or disdained for far too long. As more and more people begin to see the incomplete areas in our current medical system, especially as related to chronic, degenerative disease, a homeopathic renaissance is occurring.

Unfortunately there is a shortage of well-trained physicians to treat chronic disease. I get frustrated tell me that they have tried homeopathic remedies did not work. It always turns out that the person t was not a bona fide homeopathic physician with pro skills.

If you do seek Homeopathic treatment, it is ess a properly trained professional. Many people ar in homeopathy, yet it takes several years of dilig be able to correctly diagnose and select remedies. In m it is best if your Homeopath is a dedicated naturopatl doctor who has learned the importance of the ment symptoms in diagnosis.

Also, make sure they are familiar with the imp healthy mouth, since homeopathic treatments can be with if there are problems with the mouth and te refer your health care provider to this book. He o know at least as much as you do!

is a combination of several flowers called *Rescue Remedy*. This is extremely useful dentally to help calm an apprehensive patient. It is also very beneficial in a specific dental instance: once in a while it becomes necessary to use anesthetic with epinephrine. Sometimes a patient reacts with very rapid heartbeat and consequently fears a heart attack. Normally a dentist will just assure the patient that this is not life threatening, and in about five minutes the symptoms will pass. Administration of Rescue Remedy will alleviate the symptoms in about one minute or less.

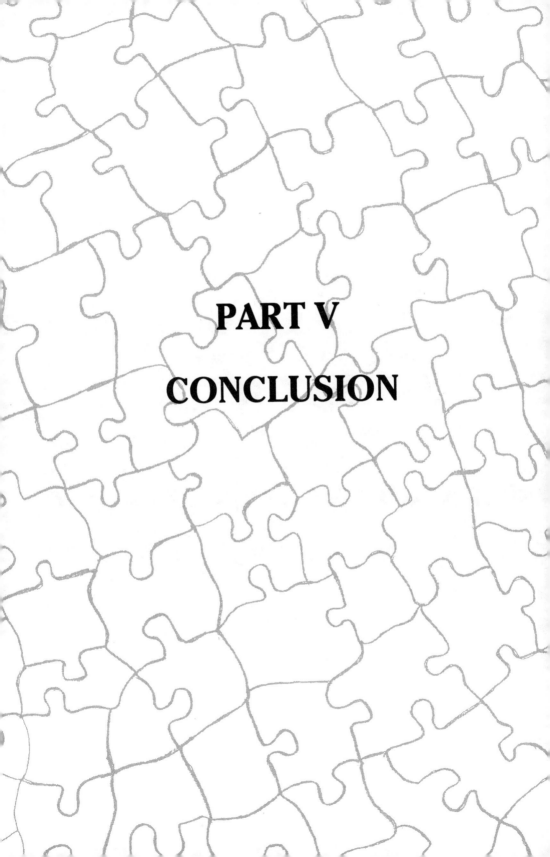

PART V

CONCLUSION

CHAPTER 29

THE FUTURE

There has always been, and will always be, a non-measurable, non-palpable something called "the art of healing." There are some things that are known, but not "known", like a thought or the soul: not known in the sense of being touchable or measurable.

This presents a problem in medicine as we know it, which is based upon Newtonian physics. The medicine of tomorrow will be based upon Einsteinian physics. We are dealing in an area where one cannot necessarily measure what is happening, because we are in the realm of energy. We are working in a non-physical dimension. Ultimately, disease comes from the mind, be that it predisposes to a pathological physical change, or the mind itself issues it into being. All natural systems of healing recognize this as being fundamental to treatment.

There are other common threads to treatment:

1. *The patient must be an active participant.* "Doctor" means teacher; it is up to the doctor or any healing practitioner to help educate the patient, in order that the patient can make the decisions regarding their treatment. Today health is more of a consumer product. The patient and/or the insurance company pay for a commodity, namely health repairs, which are to be supplied with very little input from the patient.

2. Treatment should, above all, do no harm. Much of orthodox medical/dental treatment neglects this very important tenet, either by dispensing toxic drugs on a chronic basis, or by implanting toxins in the mouth. Often more harm is done than if nothing had been undertaken. Natural therapies attempt to rid the body of toxic substances and assist the body in healing.

3. The body has a natural, innate desire to be in a state of homeostasis. The chronic use of drugs suppresses symptoms and does not act curatively. Natural therapies do not work on this suppressive level, but rather gently push and assist the body towards homeostasis.

4. A person is more than a physical being. He or she is more than can be measured by our inventions, which are extensions of our five senses - for example the microscope. A person is a spiritual, electro-dynamic, energetic, psychological being, who thinks and feels.

5. Disease is not a name; it is also not something localized which can therefore just be cut out, i.e. a cancer of the breast. The cancer which is localized to a portion of the breast is a disease of the entire person. It is a degradation of the entire immune system, or possibly a hyperfunctioning of the entire immune system. It involves not just some localized tissue, but rather the entire being, especially at the "other body" level.

6. Diet is what's eaten; nutrition is what's effective. To be effective, food must be in a form which is vibrant (vibratory). It must be full of energy, and not dead.

The future of medicine and dentistry is exciting. The use of a device like the Star-Trek Tricorder for diagnosis is on the near horizon, and one can envision the day when disease will be remedied by exposure to different vibratory waves, audible and non-audible. Imagine placing a metal implant in the mouth, and altering its electromagnetic frequency so that it can exist harmoniously within your energy field. You have a dead tooth? No problem: exposure to a certain frequency will yield it sterile, and exposure to another specific frequency will impart a new vibrational pattern, so that it does not interfere with the meridian it is on.

This is the future of Whole-Body Dentistry.

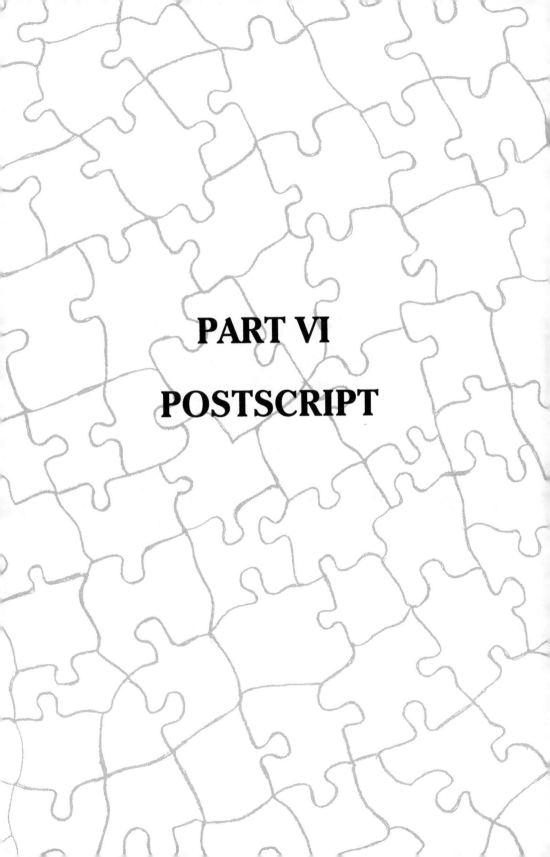

PART VI

POSTSCRIPT

PRACTICAL ADVICE FOR DENTAL WELL BEING

SELECTING A WHOLE-BODY DENTIST:

A good Whole Body Dentist should have a completely solid background in traditional dental practice and procedures, balanced by a knowledge of alternative and holistic treatments. Ideally you would want a dentist who understands the values as well as the limitations of Western medicine and who can see beyond its limited scope to help you get proper care. For example, a good Whole Body Dentist should be willing to refer patients, to traditional medical practitioners as necessary. Anyone who espouses only alterative treatments or ignores or minimizes serious symptoms that persist because they do not believe in Western medical practices is doing the patient a disservice.

Look for a dentist who is willing to take the time to work individually with each patient to determine the most important circumstances of the patient's life and stresses. Your dentist should never think in terms of standard formulas or absolutes. Everything must be evaluated in the context of the human being before them. There are no standard treatment schemes - everything is custom designed for the patient.

A good Whole Body Dentist should know and understand energetics, homeopathy, the work of Dr. Voll, the potential dangers of root canals and mercury amalgam fillings, and the steps required in safe mercury removal. He or she should also have the technical skill necessary to address these problems. Your dentist should not only be aware of these things, but should also be open and willing to discuss these practices and listen to your concerns about them. You want a practitioner who works together with, or can refer you to, a good, formally trained homeopath or naturopath. Never accept treatment from someone who just "dabbles" in homeopathy.

In addition to a medical or naturopathic physician, your dentist should also be able to work with an environmental medicine specialist, chiropractor, acupuncturist, massage therapist, or other practitioners of the healing arts to devise the most profound program of healing for you. It is essential that your dentist understands the impact of emotional states on health and the ability to heal. Equally important is an appreciation of the invasive nature of many dental procedures, with emphasis on minimizing the insult to your system. Your dentist should give a lot of attention to your health history, current overall health and nutrition - as well as explaining all treatment options thoroughly and involving you in all decisions.

Above all, you should like and trust your dentist. The personal chemistry between you and your dentist will affect your healing relationship and your ability to honestly share what is occurring in your life and health. Never minimize the importance of that relationship. If your dentist or other medical practitioner does not seem to have the time for you, ignores or discourages your questions, or in any way makes you feel uncomfortable, then you should make a change. Remember, ultimately you are responsible for ensuring your own well being. Choose your partners in health care wisely.

Brushes, Manual

There are more theories and styles of brushes to choose from than even a professional could deal with. People always ask me which toothbrush and method I advocate. Quite simply, I recommend whatever keeps your teeth clean. There is really not a lot of mystery to this process. You know that your teeth are clean when they feel nice and glassy smooth as you run your tongue against them. Just be careful to use a soft enough brush so that you do not erode the teeth or mechanically abrade the gums.

Brushes, Electric

As far as electric toothbrushes are concerned, I find they are often too rough on the teeth and mouth tissues. Some of these brushes are actually abrasive and I have noticed patients who use them can have erosion of their tooth structure. The only electric toothbrush I recommend is the Rotadent, which can be purchased through your dentist. I find it to be the most effective plaque remover with the least amount of mechanical trauma. It has a built in safety mechanism that limits the amount of pressure you can apply - if you press too hard, it stops.

Be very wary of using an electric toothbrush if you have mercury amalgam fillings. By mechanically stimulating the surface of the amalgams you increase the amount of vapor released into the oral cavity. I recently had a patient come in because after he began using an electric toothbrush he noticed that his personality began to change significantly. He was suddenly getting very angry and aggressive during his half-hour commute to work. The only reason he thought it might be vapor from the fillings was because his wife had just removed all her amalgams and experienced a phenomenal mood improvement. He stopped using the electric toothbrush and a month later, when he came in to have his amalgams removed, he related that his mood changes had improved significantly. This is also the reason that we do not polish amalgams when doing a routine cleaning of the teeth.

Brushing: Toothpaste

Toothpaste manufacturers also routinely use excessive sweeteners and even chemicals that can cause mild burning of the delicate gum tissues. If you have already read Chapter 20, then you know how dangerous fluoride can be and you are probably willing to put a little bit of effort in to track down a toothpaste without these harmful ingredients. Most health food stores now carry several brands.

My favorite brand is an herbal Tooth And Gum toothpaste. It is an excellent product; their phone number is in the appendix at the back of this book. Another option is to make your own toothpaste at home. It is really quite easy. Simply mix enough hydrogen peroxide with baking soda to make a paste, and use it as you would any other toothpaste product - but with much greater peace of mind.

Dental Floss

I do have a definite recommendation here: use unwaxed floss. When floss is coated with wax, the fibers get smoothed together resulting in less surface area to clean the teeth. Unwaxed floss is made up of many strands of fiber so there is more surface area to pick up the plaque. Some patients complain that unwaxed floss shreds. In that case, the problem is not with the floss, but with your teeth. Discuss it with your dentist. You may have a filling that is not flush with the tooth or a corroded amalgam. When flossing do not just move the floss up and down once or twice. Rub gently to remove the plaque and do each side of the tooth individually.

Disclosing Tablets

The best way to evaluate if you are consistently cleaning your teeth well is to use disclosing tablets which are available at your local drugstore. Chewing these tablets releases a harmless die which will stain any areas where plaque is forming. You can literally "train" yourself to brush your teeth properly and consistently by regularly using these tablets.

Oral pH

You can easily monitor your pH balance by purchasing saliva activated pH strips at any pharmacy, or refer to the 800 number in the appendix. Test your oral pH every morning before your first meal, and a few hours after meals. An acidic mouth with a pH below 6 is a prime breeding ground for bacteria. Your pH can be readily balanced by making changes to your diet and retesting your saliva. You will quickly learn what foods upset or restore the balance in your body. PH balance is reviewed more completely under Nutrition in Chapter 25.

Periodontal Pockets

Periodontal pockets are a breeding ground for bacteria and should be regularly cleaned out with an oral irrigator. However the typical over-the-counter irrigator has a tip that is too big to actually get into the pocket. Ask your dentist to provide you with the special needle-like rounded tips that readily slide down around the side of the tooth into the pocket. These will enable you to actually flush fluid through the pocket, breaking up and washing out bacterial colonies. The use of Tooth And Gum Tonic is an excellent irrigant.

Pregnancy

Ideally amalgam should be removed at least six months prior to conception to give the mother's body time to detoxify. This is not always feasible, of course. Amalgam fillings have also been linked to low fertility and decreased sperm motility in males, so amalgam removal in a man might be helpful for those trying to conceive. However, pregnant women should not necessarily have amalgam fillings removed during pregnancy as many adverse affects could be experienced. It is also important to be aware that amalgam removal may contribute to miscarriage in the very early stages of pregnancy. Unless they begin experiencing symptoms of mercury toxicity after becoming pregnant, it is generally best to leave their amalgams in place until after delivery.

Children

I find that the majority of children who are under the care of a homeopath experience virtually no tooth decay. This is because constitutional homeopathic treatment tends to keep the body in balance, which in turn keeps the teeth well. Of course if the child is on a diet that keeps the pH very low, they will still be susceptible to decay.

Another key factor is the mother's diet during breast feeding. The mother's nutritional intake should be optimal, in order for the baby to receive proper nourishment.

Ideally, a woman's amalgams should be removed before she becomes pregnant, because mercury passes through the placental barrier and concentrates in breast milk. If you have amalgam fillings and are concerned about breast feeding, you can ask your physician to test for high levels of mercury with a provoked urine test.

When your baby's first teeth begin to appear, it is good practice to gently wipe the teeth surfaces clean with a piece of sanitary gauze over your finger. Slowly break your children into using a toothbrush that has very soft bristles.

Never put a child to bed with a bottle of formula, juice, milk or even mother's milk. Anything other than plain water is unacceptable for a bedtime bottle because the liquid pools up against the baby's teeth and can literally dissolve them away. This is known as Baby Bottle Syndrome.

Early Dental Care

With proper eating habits, most children will not experience any problems with their baby teeth. Even though baby teeth eventually come out, they do perform vital functions. These teeth, also called deciduous teeth, are space holders for the second set of teeth and help to ensure the development of a healthy bite. Baby teeth are also critically important for proper speech development. Some baby teeth are actually still in place up to the ages of 11-15 years old. Some parents ignore decay in baby teeth because they eventually fall out. It is important, however, to have the decay removed and the tooth filled with a non-amalgam material. Those baby teeth play an important role and should be kept in good health.

When the baby teeth come in, there are often gaps or spaces between them. Parents get very upset and think that there is a problem or that dental work may be necessary. Do not worry. This is a normal phenomenon and actually serves to decrease the odds of the permanent teeth crowding.

It is good practice to have your dentist evaluate your child's bite as the permanent teeth come in. If permanent teeth are going to need orthodontics, it is better to address the problem at an early age. A good orthodontist can fit a 7 or 8-year old with a functional device that can stimulate bone growth and correct the bite with a minimum of trauma. The longer you wait, the more difficult the correction becomes.

An increasingly common dental practice for children is to apply a sealant to fill in grooves in the teeth to prevent tooth decay. This is done at an early age on the premise that bacteria can get trapped in these grooves and cause tooth decay. There is nothing wrong with sealants if they are used to fill unusually deep grooves only. But to indiscriminately seal off all the teeth as a preventative measure amounts to unnecessary dentistry.

One of the biggest problems I see with children has little to do with their teeth. They simply do not like to go to the dentist or are afraid of dentistry. This often contributes to delayed visits and poor dental care later in life.

At my office, we decided to combat this problem by instituting a "getting to know you" program for kids. Parents are encouraged to start bringing their toddlers with them during their regular dental visits. We start at around age two and a half by simply giving them a ride in the chair, letting them play with the air and water, and maybe just counting their teeth for them. This helps them get used to someone looking in their mouth and they become comfortable in the dental office, in a non-threatening manner. On subsequent visits, we may brush or clean their teeth for them, or just let them get used to the idea of dentistry.

If your dentist does not already have a program like this, ask him to provide this service for your child. These early visits can go a long way toward fostering a lifetime of good dental habits.

Children: A Knocked-Out Tooth

It is not uncommon for a child to have a tooth knocked out. If you are around when it happens, immediately put the tooth in a glass of milk. The milk replicates a nourishing environment for the cells of the tooth. There are even over-the-counter kits which have a sterile solution into which the tooth can be placed. It is a good idea to make sure your child's sports coach has these available.

Traditional dental practice would call for a root canal and re-implantation of the tooth. However, because of all the problems associated with root canal, it may be wise to consider some other options first. Children's systems are amazingly resilient and if the tooth is reimplanted as absolutely rapidly as possible, the blood and root system might simply reconnect themselves. The homeopathic remedies Arnica and Hypericum will encourage time and nature to take care of the problem. The worst that might happen is the tooth could get an abscess and cause pain in which case you would have to go back and have a BioCalex root canal.

I like to always give the body an opportunity to heal itself. This is the method I would use if it were my child and this is what I would recommend to a patient. However, I do not have any clinical experience with this procedure. Fortunately, my children never knocked their teeth out and I have not had any of my young patients lose one either. Although I have inquired, I have not been able to find a single dentist who has tried this procedure. It is not that this method would be dangerous, it is just simply because "that just is not the way its done!" Kids are so amazingly resilient that I recommend you give my option a try. Why limit nature's options?

Chipped Tooth

Thanks to modern bonding materials and techniques, a chipped tooth can be easily repaired. The missing part is simply restored with bonding. If it is a severe chip and the nerve is exposed, try not to resort to a root canal. For my patients, I would apply homeopathic calendula on the exposed nerve. I might also remove some of the nerve tissue and then cover it with a dental base material and seal it with a bonded composite. I would continue to treat it homeopathically and give it a chance to heal.

Temperature Sensitivity

Many people suddenly develop a tooth sensitivity to heat or cold. This is commonly related to a slight recession of tissue at the gum line exposing some of the underlying cementum. It will often disappear as mysteriously as it came and this is simply the body healing itself. Maintaining a proper pH balance will help to prevent occurrences and hasten healing. This type of sensitivity is sometimes also related to brushing too hard and abrading the gum tissue. In these instances, patients have gotten instantaneous relief with modified laser light treatment. Sometimes a traumatic occlusion will be the culprit and a slight adjustment of the bite, followed by modified laser light treatment, will take care of the problem.

Wisdom teeth

For a long time my philosophy on impacted wisdom teeth was to "let sleeping dogs lie." After all, if the patient was not in pain and there was no pathology present in X-rays, why do anything?

Exposure to Dr. Voll's work, and a book by Dr. Ernest Adler, **Neurofocal Dentistry,** gave me new insight into the potential problems associated with wisdom teeth. Energetically, Dr. Voll showed that the wisdom teeth are on major meridians which are connected to the heart, kidneys, small intestines, and nervous system, among others. In fact Dr. Voll felt that the area of the wisdom teeth to be the major cause of heart problems, after the fifth decade - whether from wisdom teeth themselves, or cavitations in this area.

In his book, Dr. Adler demonstrates through case histories and photos, the resolution of many recalcitrant systemic problems just from the extraction of wisdom teeth. Dr. Adler calls them "irritating thorns" that caused problems by irritation to the major nerve that runs inside your lower jawbone, called the mandibular nerve. Via feedback signal, this irritation to the mandibular nerve can create a variety of systemic reactions. Some of the problems resolved by the extraction of wisdom teeth include severe eczema, gastritis, loss of speaking voice, sciatica, heart problems, and many others.

Dr. Adler also found that the wisdom teeth did not have to be impacted to cause problems. Even when a wisdom tooth is fully erupted and in normal position, the space between the wisdom tooth and the body of the lower jawbone, called the ramus, which goes up toward the temporomandibular joint, is often inadequate. This causes stunted root development, which is evident on x-ray. Evaluation of all wisdom teeth, with EAV and neural therapy, is extremely important and must not be forgotten.

Dr. Weston Price in his nutrition studies showed that when people stopped eating their native diets, within one to two generations their jaws no longer grew as large and were unable to accommodate the wisdom teeth. Consequently, we find it increasingly common today for people to have impacted wisdom teeth.

I feel if a wisdom tooth is impacted, meaning that there is no room for it to come in, then it should be removed as soon as possible. If it can be removed before the roots are fully developed, it is an easier procedure for both the dentist and the patient. A panoramic X-ray at around age 18 will readily determine whether there are wisdom teeth and whether there is adequate room for them.

As with any extraction, I inject a homeopathic medication and also give homeopathic remedies for the patient to take orally. I treat the surgery area with modified laser light as well. These complementary therapies are often so effective that many patients need no other pain medication, and those that do, require very minimal amounts.

PART VII

APPENDICES:

ENDNOTES

1. Gerber, Richard, M.D., Vibrational Medicine: New Choices for Healing Ourselves. Santa Fe, N.M.: Bear & Company, 1996.

2. Stienman, Ralph. The Physiological Basis for Caries Susceptibility and Resistance. Journal Southern California State Dental Association, Vol XXIX, No.7, July 1961.

3. Steinman, Ralph. The Movement of Aeriflavine Hydrochloride Through Molars of Rats on a Cariogenic and non-cariogenic diet., Journal Southern California Dental Association, Vol XXXV, No. 4, April 1967.

4. Eggleston and Nylander. Correlation of dental amalgam with mercury in brain tissue. J Prost Dent. 58(6)704-707, Dec. 1987.

5. Lorscheider et al. Toxicity of ionic mercury and elemental mercury vapor on brain neuronal protein metabolism. Neurotoxicology 15(4) Twelfth International Neurotoxicology Conference. Hot Springs, Arkansas, 30 Oct-2 Nov, 1994.

6. Danscher, et al, Traces of mercury in organs from primates with amalgam fillings. Experimental and Molecular Pathology: 52:291-299, 1990.

7. Vimy, et al, Maternal-fetal distribution of mercury (203 HG) released from dental amalgam fillings. Am J of Physiology 258:R939-45, April,1990.

8. Drash, et.al, Mercury Burden of Human Fetal and Infant Tissues. European Journal of Pediatrics, 153 (8:607-610,1994)

9. "Cognitive performance of children pre-natally exposed to "Safe" levels of methyl mercury." Environmental Research,72(2): 165-72, May 1998.

10. The Coors Study, Aldolf Coors Foundation, cited in Huggins, Hal, DDS, Uniformed Consent, Charlottsville, Va: Hampton Roads Publishing, pp 66-67,1999.

ENDNOTES

11. Siblerud,R., et al, Evidence that mercury from silver dental fillings may be an etiological factor in Multiple Sclerosis. Science of the Total Environment 142:191-205, 1994.

12. Echevarria, Diana, et al, Neuro-Behavioral effects from exposure to Dental Amalgam Hg°: new distinction between recent exposure and mercury body burden. FASEB J 12:971-980,1998.

13. Lain,E.S., M.D., et al, Electro galvanic phenomena of the oral cavity caused by dissimilar metallic restoration, J ADA, vol 23 Sept 1936.

14. Ziff, Sam, et al, Dental Mercury Detox, BioProbe, P.O. Box 608010, Orlando, FL 32860

15. Meinig, George, D.D.S., Root Canal Coverup, Ojai, California: Bion Publishers, 1993.

16. From the 1983 United States Pharmacopeia Drug Information: Drug Information for the Health Care Provider. Volume 1, The United States Pharmacopeial Convention, 1982, pp. 805-807.

17. Albright, J.A., "The Effect of Fluoride on the Mechanical Properties of Bone," Transactions of the Annual Meeting of the Orthopedics Research Society, 1978, pp. 3, 98. Cited in Dr. John Yiamouyiannis, Fluoride: The Aging Factor. Delaware, Ohio: Health Action Press 1983.

18. Cordy, P.E., et al, "Bone Disease in Hemodialysis Patients with Particular Reference to the Effect of Fluoride in Sturdy of Nutritional Requirements of Patients of Chronic Hemodialysis," National Institute of Arthritis and metabolic Diseases, July 1973, pp28-59. Distributed by the National Technical Information Service of the U.S. Department of Commerce and cited in Dr. John Yiamouyiannis, Fluoride: The aging Factor, Delaware, Ohio: Health Action Press 1983.

ENDNOTES

19. Klein, Wolfgang, et al, "Biochemical Research of the Action of Sodium Fluoride on Mammalian Cells. The Effect of Biosynthesis of Nucleic Acid and Proteins of Mouse Spleen Cells In Vivo Studies,: Report of the Austrian Society of Atomic Energy , Seibersdorf Research Center, No,. 2355, pp1-10 (1974).

20. Mullenix, Phyliss, et al, Neurotoxicity of Sodium Fluoride in Rats, Neurotocicology Teratology, Vol17 No.2 p.169-177,1995.

21. Zhao, et al, Effects of high fluoride exposure on intelligence in children, Fluoride 29:4 pp 190-192, 1996

22. Tsuec, J. et al. A Food Allergy Study Utilizing the EAV Acupuncture Technique, Am Journal of Acupuncture, Vol 12 No2, April-June 1984.

23. Tucker, Dennis, Laser and Electrodiagnostic Techniques for the Isolation and Treatment of Odontogenous Foci. Am J. of Acup Vol. 18 No4, pp 345-53, 1990.

24. Rebuilding Your Patients' Health Through Free Radical Therapy, Queen and Company, Colorado Spring, CO (719)-598-4968.

25. Summers, el al, Mercury released from Dental "Silver" Filling Provokes and Increase in Mercury and Antibiotic Resistant Bacteria in Oral and Intestinal Flora of Primates. Am Society for Microbiology, April 1993, Vol 37, No.4, pp825-34.

26. Huggins, The Two Faces of Cholesterol. Chicago Dental Society Review, Vol 68. No.1, Jan 1975.

27. Heinonen, O. Dr., Dr. Demetris Albanes, on behalf of The Alpha-Tocopherol, Beta Carotene Cancer Prevention Study Group. The Effect of Vitamin E and Beta Carotene on the Incidence of Lung Cancer and Other Cancers in Male Smokers. New Engl J of Med, April 14, 1994, Vol 330 No 13, 1029-1035.

Appendix 1: Additional Reading

Atkins, Robert, M.D., *Dr. Atkins' New Diet Revolution*
Dr. Atkin's *Vita-Nutrient Solution:Nature's Answer to Drugs* - available at your local bookstore

Dispensa,Joseph, *Live Better Longer*. The Parcells Center, P.O.Box 2129, Santa Fe, NM 87504-2129. (800) 811-6784

Gerber, Richard, MD *Vibrational Medicine*, Bear & Co., Sante Fe, NM

Huggins, Hal, DDS *It's All in Your Head*
What Price Root Canals
Uniformed Consent
available at (719) 522-0566

Kaminsky & Katz, *Flower Essence Repertory* - (800) 548-0075

Levine, Barbara Hoberman, *Your Body Believes Every Word You Say*. Aslan Publishing, 2490 Black Rock Tnpk. Fairfield, CT.06432 (800) 786-5427

Null, Gary, *Get Healthy Now!*, available at your local bookstore.

Schmid, Ronald N.D., *Native Nutrition - Eating According to Ancestral Wisdom.*, Healing Arts Press, One Park Street, Rochester, VT 05767

Siegel, Bernie,M.D., *Peace, Love, and Healing*
Love, Medicine & Miracles
available at your local bookstore.

Ullman, *The Patient's Guide to Homeopathic Medicine*. (206) 233-1155

APPENDIX 1: ADDITIONAL READING

The following books can be ordered from Academy of Biological Dentistry. (831) 659-5385

> *Matrix and Matrix Regulaton* - A.Pischenger, M.D.
> *Manual of Neural Therapy According to Huneke.* P.Dosch.,MD
> *Neurofocal Dentistry* - Adler
> *Bioresonance Therapy* - Brungemann
> *Body Electric* - R. Becker, M.D.

The following books can be ordered from BioProbe, Inc. phone:(407) 290-9670; fax:(407)299-4149, www.bioprobe.com.

> *Silver Dental Fillings- The Toxic Time Bomb* - Sam Ziff
> *Mercury Poisoning from Dental Amalgam - A Hazard to
>   the Human Brain* - Patrick Stortebecker, M.D.
> *Infertility and Birth Defects - Is Mercury from Silver
>   Fillings a Hidden Cause?* Sam Ziff and Dr. Michael Ziff
> BioProbe Newsletter - to stay current on the latest scientific
> research related to the mercury/amalgam issue.

The following can be ordered from DAMS (800) 311-6265

> DAMS newsletter
> *Chronic Mercury Toxicity - New Hope* - Sam Queen
> *Beating Alzheimer's* - T. Warren

Many books on Homeopathy can be ordered from Minimum Price Bookshop (800) 663-8272

> *Organon* by Dr. Samuel Hahneman (a must read)

The following can be ordered from the Price Pottenger Foundation (800) 366-3748, (619) 574-7763, www.price-pottenger.org.

> *Dental Infections - Oral and Systemic* Vol I - Dr. Weston
> Price
> *Dental Infections and the Degenerative Diseases*, Vol II-
> Dr. Weston Price
> *Nutrition and Physical Degeneration* - Dr. Weston Price
> *Root Canal Coverup* - Dr. George Meining
> *Fluoride- The Aging Factor* - J. Yiamouyiannis

Appendix 2: Resources

Dental Referrals or Education Sources:

International Academy of Oral Medicine and Toxicology (IAOMT)

P.O.Box 628531
Orlando, FL 32860-8531
(407) 298-2450
www.iaomt.org

The Academy has a certification process, for those dentists demonstrating by written and oral examination, the fundamentals necessary for safe amalgam removal.

American Academy of Biological Dentistry
P.O. Box 856
Carmel Valley, CA 93924
(831) 659-5385

DAMS (Dental Amalgam Mercury Syndrome)

P.O.Box 64397
Virginia Beach, VA 23467
(800) 311-6265

A non-profit educational and advocacy group. Free information on dental toxins and related health issues. Doctor referrals.

Environmental Dental Association
P.O. Box 2184
Rancho Sante Fe, CA 92067
(800) 388-8124 (858)-586-7626

Foundation for Toxic-Free Dentistry

P.O.Box 608010
Orlando, FL 32860-8010

for information and referrals send a #10 sized self addressed envelope with 77cents postage attached.

Holistic Dental Association
P.O. Box 5007, Durango, CO 81301
www.holisticdental.org

Huggins Diagnostics
(719) 522-0566, www.hugnet.com

The Price-Pottenger Foundation
P.O.Box 2614, LaMesa, CA 91943-2614
(800) 366-3748,(619) 574-7763, www.price-pottenger.org

APPENDIX 2: RESOURCES

Fluoridation Education:

The Safe Water Foundation
6439 Taggart Raod
Delaware, Ohio 43015

Safe Water Coalition of Washington State
5615 W. Lyons Ct.
Spokane, WA 99208-3874
(509) 328-6704

Products or Services referred to in book:

Affinity Labeling Technologies, Inc.
235 Bolivar Street
Lexington, KY 40508
(606) 388-9445, www.altcorp.com

Testing Root-Canal Teeth

Clifford Consulting & Research
PO Box 17597
Colorado Springs, CO 80935
(719) 550-0008, www.ccrlab.com

Dental Materials Testing

Dental Herb Company, Inc.
(Herbal Toothpaste and
Mouthwash)
(800) 747-4372; (413) 582-0600

Morter Health System
(pH paper 5.5-8.0)
(800) 874-1478

Queen and Company
(719) 598-4968
www.queenhealth.com

*health consultations, seminars,
educational materials, CCN,
knowledgeable in mercury toxicity*

Natural Supplementation:

Standard Process Inc.
1200 West Royal Lee Drive
Palmyra, WI 53156
(800) 848-5061
www.standardprocess.com
*dispensed by healthcare
professionals only*

Homeopathic Detox:

HVS Laboratories
(referred to as Hoban in book)
3427 Exchange Ave.
Naples, FL 34104
(941) 643-4636, www.hvslabs.com
*dispensed by healthcare professionals
only*

APPENDIX 2: RESOURCES

Medical Sources: (for referral to physicians knowledgeable in heavy metal detoxification)

American College for Advancement in Medicine (ACAM)
23121 Verdugo Drive, Suite 204
Laguna Hills, CA 92653
(949)-583-7666, (800)-532-3688, www.acam.org

American Academy of Environmental Medicine
7701 East Kellogg, Suite 625
Wichita, KS 67207-1705
316-684-5500, www.aaem.com

American Holistic Medical Association
6728 Old McLean Village Dr.
McLean, VA 22101
(703)-556-9728, www.holisticmedicine.org

American Preventive Medical Association
9912 Georgetown Pike, Ste D-2, PO Box 458
Great Falls, VA 22066
(703)-759-0662, www.apma.net

Homeopathic Medical Resourse:
National Center For Homeopathy
801 North Fairfax St., Suite 306
Alexandria, VA 22314
(703)-548-7790, www.healthy.net/nch

Naturopathic Medical Resources:
American Association of Naturopathic Physicians
601 Valley Street, Ste.105
Seattle, WA 98109
(206) 298-0126, www.naturopathic.org

Canadian Naturopathic Association
1255 Sheppard Ave., East
North York, Ontario M2K 1E2
(416)-496-8633, www.naturopathicassoc.ca

APPENDIX 3: DETOXIFICATION BATHS

DETOXIFICATION BATHING (DETOX BATH)

SOAKING BATHS TO DRAW TOXINS OUT OF THE BODY:

Start by putting $\frac{1}{4}$ cup Baking Soda in the water for the first two weeks of detox bathing.

Soak in a tub for 10-20 minutes in water temperature that is comfortably pleasant. Take detox baths twice a week with at least a couple of days in between each bath. Continue bathing or showering as you usually would in addition to the detox baths.

After two weeks, choose from one of the following depending on how you feel.

(1) WHEN FEELING STRONG

Epsom Salt: $\frac{1}{2}$ cup to a tub of water to be used when you are feeling strong.

(2) WHEN FEELING OK (AVERAGE)

Combination: $\frac{1}{4}$ cup Epsom Salt and $\frac{1}{4}$ cup Baking Soda to a tub of water, to be used when you are feeling OK.

(3) WHEN FEELING TIRED AND FRAGILE

Baking Soda: $\frac{1}{2}$ cup to a tub of water to be used when you are feeling tired and fragile.

(4) BASIN BATHING

$\frac{1}{4}$ cup of Baking Soda or Epsom Salt in a sink of warm water. Wipe body with a wash cloth and pat dry.

AFTER YOUR BATH, SHOWER OFF USING A WASH CLOTH AND SOAP TO REMOVE ANY TOXINS THAT MAY BE ON THE SURFACE OF THE SKIN. AFTER YOUR SHOWER, PUT ON CLEAN CLOTHING SO THAT YOU ARE NOT EXPOSED TO TOXINS IN YOUR CLOTHING.

Appendix 4: Step by Step Method for Cleaning Food

PROCEDURE TO ELIMINATE SPRAYS, BACTERIA, FUNGUS, AND METALLICS
(reprinted with permission from Live Better Longer The Parcells Center 7-Step Plan for Health and Longevity by Joseph Dispenza)

Formula: Use one-half (1/2) teaspoon of CLOROX to one (1) gallon of water obtained from the usual supply. (Do Not Try to use any other product, as it will not work! Use Regular Clorox only).

Into this bath, place the fruits and vegetables that are to be treated. The thin-skinned fruits and leafy vegetables will require 10 minutes. The root vegetables and heavy-skinned fruits will require 15-30 minutes. Apples and potatoes will take 30 minutes. Timing is very important. Make a fresh bath for each group.

Remove from Clorox bath and place into a fresh water bath for 5 to 10 minutes. Now the food is ready to finish cleaning and prepare for storage. Let the food drain very well before placing it into the refrigerator.

Follow the instructions as to timing for both the Clorox bath and the rinse bath. Some are afraid that soaking the vegetables will make them lose their mineral content. This cannot happen in 15-30 minutes. The mineral activity is only increased, as you will find. You will destroy many parasites, as well as many forms of fungus found in the soil to which our bodies may become the host. It is better to be safe than sorry.

A word of caution: Do not use more Clorox than instructed, or do not leave the fruits or vegetables longer than the given time, especially the green leafy vegetables, as they will turn brown due to oxidation. There is no harm known, but the eye appeal is spoiled.

PROCEDURE FOR TREATING FOODS

Separate the foods into groups:

Vegetables:

Leafy vegetables	5-10 minutes
Root vegetables, heavy skinned or fiber vegetables	10-15 minutes

Fruits:

Thin skinned berries	5 minutes
Medium skinned fruits	10 minutes
Thick-skinned fruits	10-15 minutes
citrus fruits and bananas	15 minutes

Appendix 4: Step by Step Method for Cleaning Food

Eggs:
Eggs are at the top of our list of allergy-causing foods. This may be due to the pesticide sprays used around the pens and nests. The egg shell is porous and can absorb these poisons very quickly. Salmonella bacteria may also be present in the egg, as it is often found in the fowl. By putting the eggs through the Clorox bath for 20-30 minutes, you will find the egg has better flavor and will lose its tendency to create allergies.

Meats:
Meats are one of our heavy carriers of many toxic materials, from shots to poisons ingested in the food consumed by the animal. You will find that by placing meats in the Clorox bath, all of this will be eliminated, the flavor will be improved and the tissue tenderized. This applies to all flesh foods, including fish, which carry a heavy mercury content, and today many other toxic materials which will respond to this type of treatment, making your food more enjoyable. If your meat is frozen, you will find it will not lose its juices if placed in the Clorox bath, using the same formula. This timing would be 15-30 minutes for a 2-5 pound weight. Frozen turkey or chicken should remain in the Clorox bath until thawed. All meats should be treated in the Clorox bath with the exception of ground meats.

Benefits:
There are several advantages to this treatment. Fruits and vegetables will all keep much longer. The wilted ones will return to a fresh crispness. The faded color will vanish and the faded flavor will be gone. For your efforts, you will have fresh, crisp vegetables that will keep twice as long. The flavors of both fruits and vegetables will be greatly enhanced, tasting like they have just been taken from the garden-plus all the harmful possibilities have been removed. The dangers from these sprays and other materials used in so many ways is greater than you know.

INDEX

INDEX

INDEX

INDEX

About the Author

Mark A. Breiner, DDS, is a graduate of the Temple University School of Dentistry and has been a practicing dentist since 1971. He served as a Captain in the United States Army for two years, where he was appointed head of Dental Prosthetics at the White Sands Missile Range. In 1973 Dr. Breiner established a private practice in Fairfield, Connecticut. He was among the first proponents in Connecticut in the 1970's of dental treatment for TMJ suffers. As his TMJ patients found relief from their suffering, other seemingly unrelated complaints disappeared. This led Dr. Breiner to realize that dentistry viewed as part of the "whole person", was a missing link that needed to be explored.

Dr. Breiner is a member and Fellow of the Academy of General Dentistry; a Charter member, Board member, and Fellow of the International Academy of Oral Medicine and Toxicology; a member of the American Academy of Biological Dentistry, the Holistic Dental Association, and The National Center for Homeopathy.

Dr. Breiner has lectured throughout the country to both professional and lay audiences on Rehabilitative Dentistry, electro-dermal screening, homeopathy, and biological dentistry.

Dr. Breiner has been mercury free for over twenty years. He is currently in private practice in Orange, CT.

Dr. Breiner is available for lectures to public or professional groups. Please write or fax the publisher, Quantum Health Press, LLC.

CHECK YOUR FAVORITE BOOKSELLER
OR ORDER HERE

Please send _____ copies of **Whole-Body Dentistry**™ at $19.95 each, plus $5 shipping for first copy, $1.00 shipping each additional copy to same address. (Connecticut residents please add appropriate sales tax per book). Orders outside of the U.S. must be by credit card, additional postage to be added, if applicable.

My check for $_____ is enclosed.

Please charge $_____ to my ☐ VISA   ☐ MasterCard

Name _____

Business/Organization _____

Address _____

City/State/Zip _____

Country _____

Phone _____ Fax_____

Card # _____ Exp. Date_____

Name on Card _____

Signature _____

Please make your check payable and return to:

Quantum Health Press, LLC
P.O. Box 1637, Fairfield, CT 06432

Call your credit card order to: 888-277-1328

(Outside United States Call 203-396-0342)

Quantity Discounts Available

Call 888-277-1328

From the Patients

"I was diagnosed with Graves Disease in June of 1996 but rejected the conventional treatment of radioactive iodine to destroy the thyroid; instead I decided to research alternative medicine as a means of treatment. I discovered numerous articles on the harmful effects of mercury fillings and decided to have mine removed. Dr. Breiner removed my mercury fillings in August of 1996 and within 6 weeks my symptoms started to disappear. Six months later I was asymptomatic as verified with extensive blood tests. It is my strong belief that a cause and effect relationship precipitated this change. Today, two years later, I remain symptom free."   I. Ryan

"In 1993 I started to feel pain in a lower right molar in which I had a root canal. After a check-up and X-rays we determined that I had a very bad infection at the root of this tooth, and we decided to pull it. I made an appointment for the extraction, but before I could get there, I developed a severe case of pleurisy. I was so ill I had to postpone my dental appointment until after I got somewhat better. I had the tooth extracted about two weeks later on December 23, 1993, and all my lung symptoms immediately disappeared. I no longer had any pain or unusual sensations in my lungs. Although I was told that I might have an uncomfortable night following the extraction, I was surprised to find that I slept better than I had in 20 years, because suddenly my sinuses were completely clear, and I could breathe effortlessly all night long. This was a real bonus because having suffered from right-sided congestion and sinus headaches for many years, and having tried a number of unsuccessful treatments, I had come to believe this was something that I would live with for the rest of my life." N. Adams

From the Patients

"A real pioneer in modern dentistry. No more high blood pressure after the removal of my amalgams. Another example of holistic practices - the whole being is the sum of the parts."
J. Dresden

"As a last effort to regain my health I decided to have my seven root canal teeth extracted. As a result I now experience higher energy levels, mental clarity, and a much stronger immune system. Thank you, Dr. Breiner"   G. Fiene

"For years I visited doctors seeking the cause of increasingly debilitating health problems, which were really due to mercury poisoning. I am grateful to Dr. Breiner for his skillful diagnosis and removal of the mercury in my mouth, which allowed my body to heal completely."   K. Furman

"I was diagnosed with MS in 1994. Prior to seeing Dr. Breiner I suffered from double vision and was very dependent on my cane for balance and strength when walking. Since having my amalgams fillings removed, I haven't had my vision problems and I no longer use my cane." A. Ryczewski

"I suffered from numbness in my extremities, including my hands with random muscular "twitching". My initial diagnosis was for Carpal Tunnel Syndrome. The symptoms then spread to my feet and lower legs. Carpal Tunnel surgery was performed on my left hand, however, my symptoms worsened! Testing for MS, Lyme Disease, HIV etc. were all Negative. After amalgam removal, and nutritional supplementation, my symptoms have been in steady regression. Overall, my well-being is immensely improved."   M. Guarnieri

From the Patients

"When I first became a patient of Dr. Breiner I was at my wit's end with the problems of chronic fatigue. After having extensive metal fillings and posts (pins) removed from my mouth and detoxing with herbs and baths, my energy level rose from a two/three to an eight on a scale of one to ten. In addition, the blood test which checked dental products was of great help... I can honestly say this dental experience was the first time I left the dentist _without_ feeling sick."   K. Avery

"Chronic fatigue accompanied my multiple sclerosis for about the last six years. And even with my doubts, I decided to make an appointment (I was a strong advocate of "traditional" medicine and treatment).

After discussing my history and problems, I decided on a game plan that included removing a root canal tooth that I had received ten years ago (1988). Within 30 days, after the root canal was removed, it was apparent that I had substantially more energy! I used to go to bed at 8:00 p.m. nightly, from exhaustion, and now I am going to bed at midnight! Four additional waking hours per day, 28 additional waking hours per week, etc. It's like you've given me a whole new life.

Also, unexpectedly, after the removal of the root canal tooth, my vision improved so that I no longer wear my prescription eyeglasses! I am extremely pleased. I have a renewed lease on life and now have a new respect for alternative medicine and treatment. I am continually striving for purity in my life. I no longer blindly treat the problem but I try to treat the whole body."   R. S. Doherty

From the Patients

"I had twenty-two amalgams placed in my mouth during the summer of my thirteenth year. I immediately noticed that I had very little strength or stamina to ride my bike or run or most any other activity. By the time I was fifteen, I was severely depressed and was crying often. I have recently found out that mercury is primarily excreted in the tears. So, it was good that I cried a lot.

When I was thirty, a gold crown was placed over one of those original amalgams by a dentist who had told me that the entire crown and filling was gold. At the age of thirty-nine, a large, over-drilled amalgam filled tooth resulted in a root canal. Whatever energy I did have was now cut in half, and I developed a very "weak" back. Then, at the age of forty-four, another tooth was given a root canal. Within six months, I had a ruptured disc. I now had experienced severe back pain for six years. My health declined rapidly. I became hypothyroid, hypoadrenal, hypoglycemic, had systemic candida, had developed numerous food metabolic intolerance, chronic fatigue syndrome and memory loss. It was difficult for me to articulate speech. I had put on thirty pounds in three years, and my blood pressure was 144/90.

My first procedure by Dr. Breiner was the removal of all the simple amalgams, that is, not crowns or root canal fillings. I expected to have improved health over the next year. Instead, the improvement was dramatic and immediate. I felt as if thirty-five years of stress and pain was draining from my body right in the dentist's chair. Two days later my blood pressure was 112/76! Over the next nine months, I had every crown replaced, and had all two root canal teeth pulled out, and a cavitation from an extracted wisdom tooth cleaned out. With each procedure, I could actually see and feel my body healing, especially in my spine. My body's ability to heal after straining was that of a teenager, about one to three days. Previously, it would take me months to heal. I was now not severely stressed by noise as I used to be. Also, I love to smile now, my teeth look beautiful!"

B. A. Burke, R.PH., M.S.